RELENTLESS METTLE

My Cancer, My Rules

By Stephen Brown

Foreword by Dave Scott

ISBN: 978-1-329-60435-3

First Edition

Table of Contents

Dedication

This is dedicated to all cancer warriors everywhere and to their extremely critical and sometimes overlooked support teams. While fighting this fight can be a challenge, there is safety, security, and strength in our numbers. To those warriors who have lost their battle, we will continue this fight in your name and in your honor. We will relentlessly push on until we find the cures.

Foreword

My involvement with The Leukemia & Lymphoma Society's Team in Training program started in 1999. I was aware of Team in Training's impact in the running community and several people approached me with the concept of starting a triathlon program. I became immersed into TNT and LLS to learn more about the blood cancer community and the profiles of the many people impacted by blood cancers. This led to incredible opportunities to work with people like Steve Brown, as I learned more about all of the wonderful work that TNT and LLS were doing. I saw so many patients reaching remission from their disease as a result of these efforts. This provided a wonderful sense of satisfaction and fulfillment for me as the national coach.

I have been able to connect with numerous patients such as Steve who was diagnosed with chronic lymphocytic leukemia in 2006 and who has fought through a couple of

relapses since his initial diagnosis and I am amazed at the
positive approach and outlook he has sustained throughout
his journey when his future may have appeared at times
uncertain. When I hear stories such as Steve's, I am
amazed at the irony of how positive people can be. I never
sensed a forlorn feeling from Steve and his positive and
upbeat outlook has had an infectious effect on so many of
the people that he touches.

I am grateful for having had the opportunity to work with
Team in Training and The Leukemia & Lymphoma Society
over the years and network with so many patient athletes,
bearing witness to the adversity they have had to overcome.
I have had the good fortune of being a very healthy guy so I
haven't had to personally deal with the physical and
emotional impacts of such a disease. I honestly don't know
if I would have had the intestinal fortitude to respond the
same way as Steve and so many others have.

I know Steve Brown has always taken his definition of
health very seriously, having had a great soccer career and
decades of success in the sport of triathlon prior to his
diagnosis. But through his disease he has found a way to
continue to thrive and help others in the process. My hat is

off to Steve and all of the folks I have been lucky enough to interact with through the years in this community.

Continued health, success, and best wishes,

Dave Scott

Acknowledgements

I believe we are all the products of every experience and personal exchange that we have encountered in our lives. I know that may be a little too much to digest and you may or may not agree with me. But think about all of the people who have touched you in some way through the years. While we remember most of the people who have had an obvious influence on our lives, the truth is that many of those experiences were subtle and we may not have even realized that they were meaningful at the time. Therefore many of these game changing experiences are long since forgotten and unrecognized.

There are many people and events that I have to thank for where I am in my life today. While I can't thank them all here now, I can call out a few. First and foremost I need to thank God for giving all of us the strength and resolve to not only "get through this" but to thrive and flourish in the face of adversity. I have an incredible sense of love, pride, and joy for my wife, daughters, and now grandchildren which cannot be measured or even articulated. To them, I say thank you. I'm a lucky guy. I feel blessed in that I look at every day as an amazing gift and just when I think things can't get any better, they do.

I grew up in a pretty traditional household with two parents who were very loving and involved with everything I did. They seemed to strike a wonderful balance of being there without smothering or controlling me. They let me be a kid and find my way but with the understanding that a safety net would always be there. They allowed me to grow and be and fully supported me. While we lost my dad in 2005, my mom is alive and well and will soon turn 90 years old. To them, I say thank you.

Coaches, mentors, and teachers have always played a huge part in my life. I remember every single one and try to keep in touch with as many of them as possible. I remain in regular contact with a few coaches and teachers I had in high school and college. I owe them and want them to know they were and are still appreciated. To them, I say thank you.

My circles and networks are quite large. I like to call myself a people broker because I love connecting like minded people from all over in an effort to combine forces and shrink this oversized planet a little bit. To this day I talk to friends from my old neighborhood that I grew up with playing in the streets and playgrounds of Ardmore Pennsylvania. Some of these friendships date back to kindergarten and first grade. There is no doubt that those relationships formed so long ago, have helped define me. To each and every one of them, I say thank you.

Given the fact that I live with a chronic form of leukemia, I would be remiss if I didn't acknowledge and openly express my gratitude for the many health care professionals who have played a part in my diagnosis, treatments, and ongoing care. We are lucky to have the resources that we have and to all of them, I say thank you.

Introduction

This collection is the intersection of my cancer experiences, my multisport lifestyle, and my overall outlook on life. Call it the intersection of parallel lines if you will. When you sit in a recliner in a chemotherapy suite for several hours, your mind has a tendency to go places. Some of those places have been captured here. I made a very early decision and commitment to live my experiences and my story quite publicly. I wanted to be a voice and I wanted to lead by example.

While no two individuals or cancer stories are exactly the same, I'm always happy to share my experiences and thoughts on the specifics of my own personal journey. I've learned over the years that people do really want to know, and many are afraid to ask, or they don't know who to ask. As a result of being so open with my story, I have been able to connect with so many fellow cancer warriors and their families. That's vindicating. I want patients and their families to take comfort in reading these pages and I hope they resonate hope and possibility and help people to understand they are not alone.

This is not a "how to" guide for living with cancer. But my hope is that it will provide a source of comfort and inspiration for somebody out there. These are some of the details of my experience including perspective from my wife and kids. Consider this recommended reading for an unknown journey you are about to embark on.

I've learned a few things in my 25 years of racing and almost 9 years of living with a chronic leukemia. That equates to 26 full marathons, an ultra marathon in South Africa, 11 ironman triathlon finishes, countless shorter races.... and ...46 visits to the chemotherapy suite. Lessons tend to come out of that kind of stuff. And I will continue to learn and build both relationships and experiences as time rolls on.

Rewind

I received my calling into the world of endurance sports in 1986 when a friend invited me to do a triathlon with him. I scrambled to borrow a bike and a helmet and had no idea what else to wear but was instantly drawn in and addicted to what I saw on race day. I couldn't quite put my finger on what made these people tick, but I knew I wanted to be one of them.

I continued racing shorter races but it wasn't too long before I worked my way up to marathons and eventually ironman triathlons. I was healthy. I was happy. And I felt like I was setting good examples of healthy living for my kids who came to so many of my races and crossed so many finish lines with me. That was my lifestyle for 20 years. –And it was a good one. But we live in a world of perpetual change, often unaware of what may lie ahead.

2005 proved to be a very challenging year. My father had a large tumor removed and spent two months in intensive care as a result of complications from the surgery. We were at that hospital nearly every day and sadly we lost him in August of 2005. Still grieving the loss of my dad, yet attempting to usher in the Christmas spirit, my mom was rushed to the very same hospital needing triple bypass and aortic valve replacement surgery. That valve needed to be replaced a second time within days as it was malfunctioning. This meant two open heart surgeries within days for my then 80 year old mother. Somehow, that surgery and her subsequent recovery were successful. But it was an emotionally draining period of time. We were ready to flip the calendars to 2006 and embrace the New Year with renewed hope.

In early 2006 I started having difficulty swallowing. This worsened to the point of having trouble simply swallowing anything at all. I tried a number of things to try to treat these symptoms, but nothing seemed to give me any sustained relief. Eventually, I saw an ear, nose, and throat doctor who immediately ordered a tonsillectomy. That was not how I wanted to spend my 46th birthday but I was willing to accept the surgery if it was going to resolve the problem. In preparation for surgery, I needed to have preoperative blood work drawn and this is where the slope got slippery. I received a phone call a few days prior to the scheduled surgery and was told that my tonsillectomy would need to be put on hold. There had been a problem detected in my blood work and I was advised to consult an oncologist.

Cancer. It happens. It happened to me. On February 24th 2006 my wife and I sat in the office of an oncologist who we had just met and tried to process what he was telling us. I had chronic lymphocytic leukemia ("CLL"). This would require several weeks of chemotherapy and then two years of follow up treatments. And even that wouldn't "cure" the disease as it is a chronic blood cancer that would need to be lived with and managed. This diagnosis came out of the blue. My initial and desperate thought was that some sick person's chart clearly must have been mixed up with mine. It wasn't. The chart was mine and I was that sick person.

My perspective on cancer was always that it was something that happened to others. An athlete like me doesn't get sick. I was an Ironman, several times over. I grew up one of those active kids who played every sport that I could sink my teeth into. I attended college on a soccer scholarship. I hung on the fringe of a pro soccer career and then played semi professionally for a number of years. I lived clean and healthy. So I assumed that I of all people should get a free pass on disease like cancer. I was wrong.

So with every possible emotion spiraling in a mad freefall, I began the first of four one week long rounds of chemotherapy at our local hospital. I hit some physical and emotional dark patches but they certainly weren't all dark. These patches were cyclical and interspersed with rays of hope and positivity. Things got better. My tolerance to the treatment drugs improved and I started showing signs of progress. By the 3rd round my blood counts were slowly returning to normal and I had reached my first remission.

We made a party out of chemo whenever we could. We made it an event. My wife came to every treatment. My daughters occasionally skipped school to come hang out with us and we would often all eat lunch together in the chemo suite. And I always needed to try to be the class clown to add a little levity to the situation. But that's who I am in almost any situation.

As I reconciled everything that I was experiencing, I made a few key decisions that both kept me sane and at the same time changed my life. One was to practice the simple adage of controlling the things I could control. I couldn't control the diagnosis. But I could control a lot of how I reacted to that diagnosis. In that respect, my thought process was exactly the same as it is on race day. I drew many parallels between the challenges I was facing with the disease and the challenges we all face in sport, and in life.

Within days of my diagnosis, I signed on as a triathlon coach with The Leukemia & Lymphoma Society's Team in Training program. Through this program, I get to train aspiring and veteran triathletes who are in turn raising funds and awareness for my blood cancer. It has been a magical partnership and I have been blessed to meet and work with some incredible people through the years. The Leukemia & Lymphoma Society has funded many breakthrough therapies in the global fight against blood cancers and provides many crucial resources to patients and their families. At the center of all of this, is Team in Training. They have truly become a second family to me.

Another critical decision I made was to remain in motion. I have learned through the years that I am always happiest when I am moving. I've never known if I am running towards or away from something, but when I am moving, I am whole. It is more than just a way to stay in shape. It is how I have always coped and it is my therapy. So I held onto that and kept up my training through my treatments – often running home from chemo. I made it part of a game. I challenged the disease back and made up some of my own rules of engagement.

The combination of effective drugs, a great medical team, an amazing support crew, and a good mindset allowed me to remain in some kind of shape while beating cancer. I was fortunate in that I was able to race and train throughout my diagnosis and subsequent treatments. Shortly after my first round of treatments, I was back to racing again and seven months post diagnosis I raced the Chesapeakeman Ultra distance triathlon as race director and good friend Rob Vigorito proudly and with much emotion dubbed me "RemissionMan".

Through Her Eyes

As told by Mary Grace Brown.

In 2005, we had an extremely difficult year. Steve's dad was experiencing increased shortness of breath and after being evaluated, he was found to have a very large tumor in his right lung. An 8 pound tumor was removed, and Dad did well immediately post operatively, but had many subsequent infections and spent all but one day in the ICU at Bryn Mawr Hospital between June 8th and August 5th.

Steve had a heart to heart talk with Dad, saying he would dedicate his 2005 Ironman race in Lake Placid, NY to him, and wore his WWII dog tags during the race. This particular race was difficult for Steve but we all just assumed it was due to the troubling summer and interrupted training schedule. We would later learn that his race challenges were actually something related to his health.

A few weeks after returning from Lake Placid, Dad passed away. A few months after that, Steve's mom went into congestive heart failure and needed coronary artery bypass surgery and a mitral valve replaced. The mitral valve was replaced twice. The whole family was exhausted come 2006 and looked forward to a new year of healing.

Steve had a recurring enlarged tonsil problem and was treated with Prednisone tapering doses and antibiotics on and off for a couple years. Finally, after months of the tonsils touching and impeding Steve from swallowing even peanut butter & jelly sandwiches, Steve thought he would have them removed. We went to the ear, nose & throat specialist who agreed that they needed to come out. Steve thought he would have the surgery at a time when triathlon training was slower, so a February surgery was planned.

I will never forget where I was when I got the call from Steve saying that the doctor called him and said, "Mr. Brown there is a problem with your blood work. You need to see a hematologist oncologist."

I was driving by Delaware County Memorial Hospital in Drexel Hill Pennsylvania at the time of the call. I thought to myself, "He has an infection! He needs to get to the hospital!" I called the oncology practice at DCMH and was able to make an appointment for Steve with Dr. Stephen Shore the next day. I called our primary care physician and asked if Steve should get to the hospital. He said, "No, but keep the appointment with Dr. Shore."

We were in disbelief that it could be anything but an infection, which after blasting with antibiotics; he could have the surgery and get on with life.

Our daughters were in high school at the time. We wanted to keep them in the know, but first needed to find out for ourselves what this was. The first meeting with Dr. Shore was a whirlwind. He evaluated Steve, and his blood work, and gave his initial thoughts of a chronic lymphocytic leukemia diagnosis. This, of course would need to be confirmed with a CT scan, a bone marrow biopsy, and further blood work. Steve was amazing during these tests. As a nurse, I thought, no problem - I can handle being with Steve during the bone marrow biopsy. Dr. Shore was very tuned in to my feelings. He saw I was getting queasy and invited me to leave the exam room and get something to drink in the office kitchen. I felt horrible that I could sit with patients in the hospital during such a procedure, but I couldn't with my own husband. Dr. Shore assured me that it is different when it is your family member and not your

*patient. I appreciated how Dr. Shore and the whole staff at
his office treated us with such care.*

*At one point, however, Dr. Shore told Steve he would have
to put 'all that training and intense exercising aside'. Steve
assured the doctor that if he took away his fitness regimen
he would be dealing with a lot more than just leukemia. It
was nice to see that Dr. Shore was able to meet Steve in the
middle and encouraged him to listen to his body for cues as
to when to rest and when to work out. On a funny note,
when Dr. Shore asked Colleen at his office to schedule his
diagnostic tests, he told Colleen that Steve spells Stephen
the right way....with a 'PH'. That's something that Steve
has always been very adamant about. His name is NOT
spelled with a 'V'. My husband and Dr. Shore had and
continue to have a wonderful way of communicating and
sharing a laugh at just the right times.*

*The day Steve and I met with Dr. Shore for the official
diagnosis was February 24th. All test results led to a
chronic lymphocytic leukemia diagnosis. We were able to
somewhat prepare for this through the week, but hearing
the confirmation news was tough. We went ahead and
scheduled the chemo treatments. Dr. Shore told Steve that
this disease is not common in people Steve's age, and there*

isn't a lot of data available to give an estimation of survival rates. Steve assured the doctor that he would set the bar for future estimation rates at a high level. He was determined to beat this.

Leaving the office, we looked at each other and asked, "Now what?" I said, "Let's go see Dad." There is a bench overseeing the playground at the Veterans Memorial Park in Broomall Pennsylvania that was dedicated to Dad's honor. Steve was able to sit on the bench, stare at the bench, walk around the bench, walk around the park and I did my best to keep up with him with my short legs. He turned around and hugged me - I cried - he said, "I feel worse for you that you are going to go through this". Wow - for him to say that made me cry harder. What a special moment. He didn't think of himself, but for me. Then Steve ran fast and hard up a steep hill in the park and let out a huge battle cry. He came down and we hugged again, saying we were ready to do this together. And the next plan was to tell our daughters Jennifer and Danielle.

We picked up the girls at Upper Darby High School. They suspected something when Steve and I both showed up. I was a visiting nurse and had some flexibility in my work day. So it was common for the girls to see me, but not both of us. Steve worked in Delaware and was rarely around at that time of the day.

We rested on the couches at home and Steve, in his very positive, very upbeat way, told the girls he had a blood condition that needed treatments - he was not sick, but had a condition that needed treatment. The girls looked to me and said; now you can tell us what this is. They knew it would come a little more realistic from me, given I work in healthcare. I told them the condition is leukemia - which is a cancer they both stated. I agreed, and also emulated Steve's commitment to fighting this and staying positive. Jennifer and Danielle had a look of 'deer in headlights' about them and needed to process the information, but they also decided to follow Steve's lead and stay positive during his fight. I was so proud of them and how they rallied behind Steve. There were tearful moments, of course, but they were so strong.

We next told Steve's Sister Chris, who immediately stopped over with a bottle of Merlot. Then we talked to Steve's mom, as well as my parents and then had a meeting with my siblings. I am the last of 7 Snyder children. My brothers and sisters decided to have a combination birthday and cancer fighting party, as Steve's chemo was to start the next day. It was a great day of feeling united, supporting Steve and resolving to fight this together.

I bought Steve a laptop for his birthday, initially because I knew the original 'tonsillectomy' surgery would have driven him crazy and the laptop would give him the opportunity to journal and continue to write for the online triathlon magazine he was involved with. He reached out to his long time race director friend, Rob Vigorito, and brought him up to speed. Rob was connected with some prominent physicians at the University of Maryland's School of Medicine who took a look at Steve's blood work and confirmed that the treatment plan for Steve was appropriate. Rob was so instrumental in helping Steve with this new challenge. It seemed like triathletes came out of the woodwork and reached out to Steve. I heard Steve say that they told him he had very long tentacles in the community he doesn't even know about.

One day Steve opened his laptop to Rob's website and saw the Leukemia & Lymphoma Society Team in Training logo and had his 'ah hah' moment. He reached out to the local chapter's triathlon coach, Todd Wiley, whom he knew and looked up to as an amazing triathlete. Todd welcomed Steve into the LLS TNT family of coaches and Steve has been helping train triathletes ever since. I will never forget the first practice Steve attended. He was tearful when he came home, stating how he is helping people reach their fitness goal of completing a triathlon, while they were raising money to fight his cancer. It was such a wonderful feeling. "A win-win situation".

During treatment, Steve had many phone calls, emails, and visits from people in all areas of his life: family, childhood friends, fellow athletes, college buddies, neighbors, all showing their support. Steve decided early in treatment that he would take control and run home from chemo to show cancer that it cannot win. He used visualization imagery techniques such as imagining the cancer cells falling off his back as he ran away from them, leaving them in the dust. Steve was smart on the days he didn't feel well or had a fever, and let me drive him home on those days (and I was thankful). Our daughters went to high school right next door to the chemo suite and they made sure to visit on chemo days. We were pretty sure they were skipping classes to do so, but there was no stopping them anyway. They added so much laughter and fun and the nurses made them feel right at home. Every now and then they would ask me his prognosis, but I could only honestly answer them *that this is chronic, there isn't a cure yet, and we have to make the best of what we have.*

One evening we had a visit from my cousin Sharon and her husband John. They sat quietly and prayed. Holding hands, we truly felt the presence of Jesus Christ in the room, channeling through our bodies. Even our dog, Chelsea, had an unusual calmness about her. We sat and listened to very moving stories of faith and how Christ worked through people to bring about healing in many circumstances. It was a moving, life changing visit. Shortly after their visit, one of the enlarged glands in Steve's abdomen reduced in size - and this was one of the more stubborn ones.

Our brothers and sisters brought dinners to the house on the long chemo days. My brother Johnny was a school teacher in Philadelphia and his students wrote cards to "Mr. Steve" that were both touching and funny. One of the cards read, "I'm glad you didn't get dead". We could only laugh at that but were moved by the sentiment that this child wanted the best for Steve. "Mr. Steve" was then included in the daily prayer at Johnny's school.

Many people prayed for Steve, Jennifer, Danielle and me. These were so appreciated, and got us through. I truly believe prayer is so powerful and can get you through the toughest of times and situations. We were so thankful for our faith and the faith of others in helping us cope.

Steve was given the awesome news after 3 months of treatment, that he hit remission. We were so thrilled! Steve asked for the 4th month of treatment to be skipped all together but we were assured it was necessary to keep the leukemia at bay. We started a little happy dance outside the doctor's office that day. And we still do it after each visit before taking the stairs (NOT the elevator) back down 5 flights to the

lobby.

Steve participated in a short distance triathlon in June, and then a full iron distance triathlon in September of that year. WHAT?!!! He had chemo in June and then did an iron distance triathlon in September? YES! And the family was present at the finish line after Steve completed the 2.4 mile swim, 112 mile bike and 26.2 mile run. The race director, Rob Vigorito, gave Steve the new name REMISSIONMAN. Not a dry eye was at the finish line, or at the awards brunch the day after.

For the following two years Steve had to take maintenance treatments for one week every six months. In 2012, the leukemia decided to show symptoms in Steve and he was again treated and back in remission. In 2013 he had another need for treatment rounds and responded well. When the symptoms first returned, we were understandably sad. It felt like a thousand punches in the stomach. We thought that there was a good chance this wouldn't come back. But we are so thankful that there are treatments for this, that there are newer drugs being discovered every day, and that doctors and nurses know exactly what to do and how to help Steve fight this.

We have learned over the past 9 years how a diagnosis as horrible as cancer can pull people together in such loving, positive ways. Our friends and families are there for us at all of our fundraisers, and come up with creative ways to help raise money for the Leukemia & Lymphoma Society, as well as organizations such as the Livestrong Foundation, Headstrong Foundation, and the Team Inspiration Community – who are all committed to finding cures.

Steve knows how much cancer 'sucks' and living with it can be so hard at times, but he looks at it as a blessing in a way. This experience has brought so many people together in a positive way with a good goal, leaving a feeling of connection and love. He often speaks to large groups and talks about how people get 'stuff' and it is important how you react to the 'stuff' so you don't give it the power. Steve also is trained to outreach to people who are newly diagnosed with leukemia or lymphoma. I usually know when he disappears into another room to call someone, and when the call is finished, Steve has such a look of peace about him. Helping other people really gives him joy. It is his chocolate.

As hard as it may be at times, it is difficult to find a real reason to complain. I have a super positive, super energetic, super loving, super crazy (at times), super relentless husband who will not let this bring him down. This has bonded us closer than ever. He made it easier for us. And so did the grace and blessings from our relentless God.

Through Their Eyes

As told by Danielle Brown and Jennifer Schoener

My dad is a very charismatic guy. He's a creative and inspirational writer and speaker who is rarely at a loss for what to say, or how to say it.

That's why it was weird when he sat my sister and me down to give us his "tonsillitis" update. He didn't have many words that day... and he wasn't quite as eloquent as usual. There were long pauses and there was tension, yet somehow he was calm and seemed confident.

I'll be honest. Looking back I have no idea what he said or how he said it. I know he said everything would be all right; but can you really focus after that point? When you hear "everything will be just fine" ... well the rest is just a blur. I did, however, pick up on one key word- leukemia.

His "tonsillitis" was not tonsillitis ... it was a much nastier word.

I had a thousand thoughts. More than that actually.

So let me get this straight. My former semi-professional soccer playing, iron distance triathlon racing father has cancer? That can't be true. He trains, he eats right, he does the right things and everyone loves him. He's strong, athletic and indestructible. Cancer happens to people in movies and on the news... it happens to other people. Far away people. Cancer patients look sickly. For someone who never had a close relationship with a cancer patient- that's how it seemed anyway. As a high school sophomore girl with priorities all over the place, I was given quite the reality check. I didn't get it. I questioned everything and started to realize that anything could happen. Cancer doesn't discriminate and there are some situations that you just can't rationalize or explain. This was tough.

My dad can make any crappy situation okay, but this wasn't just a crappy situation. News that seemed like a mountain to me, was merely a bump in the road for him. I admired him for that. The way he reacted to his cancer diagnosis was nothing short of inspirational and maybe even a little crazy. I think he took about five "woe is me"

minutes before jumping into "this won't stop me" mode.
Five minutes. I think I would have taken more than that…

Now I won't go into long details about his journey to
recovery. He will tell you more about that. I will tell you
that my father impresses me every day of my life. I admire
the way he grabbed his diagnosis by the horns and refused
to let it bring him down. I admire the way he took his
disease and turned it into something beautiful through
fundraising and helping others, even if it wasn't always
easy. I believe his positive attitude was as powerful and
influential in his recovery as the drugs were. His character
never swayed and his perspective stayed strong. It wasn't
long before my family decided to stop being afraid and
start focusing on how we can help him crush cancer.

He is now a resource for those going through similar
situations. People look to him for positivity and hope.
People admire his journey and reach out for affirmation
that things can and will be okay.

This ongoing journey with him keeps me in check. Just
knowing him reminds me that I can turn any situation
around and find the silver lining. He reminds me on my
most dramatic of days that perhaps spilling coffee down a
new shirt or running late for work are far from the worst

things that could happen in the world. 1 couldn't ask to
know a better guy. **- Danielle Brown**

***

I'll never forget being sat down by my parents in my senior
year of high school to talk. "Wait what? Did you just say
Daddy has cancer?" Before then, the words coming out of
my parents mouths felt so far away. Chemotherapy,
Cancer, Leukemia, this was the stuff of nightmares. What
made it more confusing to me was the sense of calm I
picked up from my dad.

This was unfamiliar territory to us, and I was just a kid
trying to read my parents the best I could to help me decide
how I felt about the situation. My dad was eerily calm, my
mom was supportive. Maybe it was because he always
promised me he would live to be 200 years old. I'm positive
he had gone through (and maybe was still going through)
an internal freak out, but his attitude during that talk would
never give that away. He was ready to fight. Was I? Could I
even be that brave? No it wasn't my fight, but was I ready
for his? Could I watch my dad be "sick" and actually be
helpful versus a big blubbering ball of panic? These were
the selfish thoughts I had to work through as I did fast

walking laps around our block attempting to make sense of it all.

So in trying to find clarity, I realized that the person who's always made the most sense to me to this day is my dad. I headed back to the house ready to adopt his positive attitude so we could all eventually, with long hours of treatment and care, put this whole mess behind us. I chose to believe this diagnosis would be good somehow, and I did that because of my dad's strength. I think we all fed off of each other that way, and still do. We needed to stick together as a family like always, this was no different. When I chose to believe in the good, I had no idea just how good it could be.

Let me be clear, cancer sucks. But what my dad has been able to do with it and in the face of it blows my mind, and has helped shape me into the person I am today. I've learned so much about my dad, about resilience and positivity, about how to consistently turn bad to good and just how much the mind influences the body. I've learned about unpredictability, and the power of a good plan. I've learned a lot about how to help people and how to let people help you; the full circle lifestyle that was never more prevalent in my dad's world was and is awe inspiring.

I carry all of this with me, and I know that in the face of anything I can be that person too. Cancer sucks, but I'm lucky to have a dad that can scold it on multiple occasions, and then turn it around and use it to help so many people. Cancer is an ongoing fight for him and affecting positive change through that is an ongoing choice, but because of his courage I know that all that means is he still has AT LEAST 146 years to inspire people. After all, he promised me 200. - **Jennifer Schoener**

Club Membership

So you've just been diagnosed. Or perhaps the diagnosis of a friend or a loved one has brought you here. Whatever brought you here doesn't matter, I'm glad you are.

Diagnosis is scary. Disease is scary. Treatments are scary. And our own mortality is the scariest of all. But there truly is safety in numbers. There are a number of excellent patient resource groups and services that are available and I encourage you to ask your doctor for a good listing of resources and educational materials. Visit only recommended and approved websites, and please, under no circumstances, should you take off on a wild Google search mission to try to become an expert on your disease. I made that mistake.

Another mistake that many newly diagnosed patients make is to try to wrap their arms and head around every detail, every nuance, and every possible option, and outcome while only half listening to a doctor explain their situation. They are half listening because there is an even louder voice in their head telling them they are probably going to die. (And the odds are the doctor never even uttered those words or anything close to them).

I know it's a scary situation and uncharted territory but it's really important to try to relax, ask questions of your medical team (many times if need be), and take your journey one small step at a time. Dissect it to the smallest manageable bite that you can emotionally process and work on meeting each hurdle one at a time. Don't lose track of the big picture, but don't become so consumed with the enormity of your diagnosis that it prevents you from celebrating the small victories along the way. You need those wins. And your spirit needs to celebrate them.

Be in control but trust the experts. Your illness is new to you but not to them. Believe in them and let them do what they have been trained to do.

It's normal to go through the initial "why me" phase. Everyone does. But it's critical to your success that you build that bridge and find a way across it. Assess the situation. Understand the path forward. Commit to getting well.

You have cancer. Attack back. Cancer can be beaten.

CLL Defined

When my doctor first uttered the words chronic lymphocytic leukemia to me, I will be the first to admit that I tuned out two thirds of what he said. As we sat in his office and discussed the details I heard a lot of things I didn't quite understand, coupled with a few things that I didn't think could possibly even apply to me, coupled with the racing thought of "when can I get the hell out of this office?!?" Of course I eventually learned more than a little about the disease, the various treatments available, and what the typical patient profile looked like. I also learned that I was about as atypical as atypical can be.

Keeping the definition simple, consider my cancer a bunch of unorganized and undeveloped white blood cells with no inherent function in the world other than to get in the way. I'm not kidding. But I'll provide a little more detail as found on the Leukemia & Lymphoma Society's website.

Chronic lymphocytic leukemia (CLL) results from an acquired (not present at birth) change (mutation) to the DNA of a single marrow cell that develops into a lymphocyte. Scientists do not yet understand what causes this change. Once the marrow cell undergoes the leukemic change, it multiplies into many cells. CLL cells grow and survive better than normal cells; over time, they crowd out normal cells.

The result is the uncontrolled growth of CLL cells in the marrow, leading to an increase in the number of CLL cells in the blood. CLL takes different forms. Some people have disease that is slow growing. People with minimal changes in their blood cell counts (an increase in the number of blood lymphocytes and little or no decrease in the number of red cells, normal neutrophil and platelet counts) may have stable disease for years and not even need any treatment. Other people with CLL have a faster-growing form of the disease—the CLL cells accumulate in the bone marrow and blood, and there is a significant decrease in the numbers of red cells and platelets.

I probably fall somewhere in the middle. My CLL is slow moving, but my symptoms were prevalent enough to warrant treatment. And while today there is no known silver bullet or magic pill against this type of leukemia, there are a number of very viable and effective treatment options, with several more in the development and approval pipeline.

So, like I said: consider my cancer a bunch of unorganized and undeveloped white blood cells with no inherent function in the world other than to get in the way.

The Journey Begins

As I settled in for my very first chemo treatment, I felt good. Mary Grace was with me. I was comfortable and confident. I was eager to get started only so I could put this entire thing behind me. My first day and entire first week of chemo was relatively ok. I will even call it "good" by chemo standards. We showed up, I got poked, prodded, and pumped up with a smorgasbord of supplemental drugs to offset the actual chemo side effects, as well as the chemotherapy drugs themselves. As is my nature, I tried to be as snarky as I could and make as many goofy comments as possible, and then we went home. No real nausea or extreme fatigue.

During the week I felt ok. However, after a full week of that stuff, I did start to get a little fatigued and nauseated.

But the feelings were very fast moving. I would wake up with enough energy to build a house. This was from the lingering effects of the steroid Decadron which was used to help offset the chemo side effects. Eventually I would fade out and need to take a nap. Then I would wake up again and feel well enough to work out a little or be productive in some way. It was a predictable and cyclical process that I became familiar with and adapted to. I'm convinced that staying active helped dilute all of those chemo side effects, and even helped deliver them more effectively throughout my system.

I ran home from my treatments almost every day and had self talks along the way, reminding myself and the cancer that I intended to kick the crap out of it. At times I scratched my head in disbelief that a thing like cancer had chosen to invade me. I wouldn't call it fear as much as confusion. The fact that I ran home from chemo had the nurses scratching their heads as well. But that was also part of my master plan. My hope was that if the nurses were confused, then so too was the cancer. I wanted to prove to it that I was not able to be rattled and refused to be "sick". It was another way of remaining in charge and controlling the things that I was able to control.

A few days after concluding the initial round of chemo I had a follow up doctor appointment. The moment of truth I thought. I was eager to see what kind of results this toxic exercise had yielded but I was nervous at the same time. What if it hadn't worked? What if I had pumped all of that poison in me and we didn't get the desired result? I didn't know what to expect, so I tried to keep my expectations a little low. My pre-chemo WBC was between 60,000-70,000. (The norm being 5,000 – 10,000) I almost fell out of chair when my post chemo count had dropped to 14,500. And equally as important, my RBC and platelets were still in a safe range: as was everything else for that matter. So, this stuff had done an outstanding job and I didn't appear to have suffered any breakdown or destruction of any of my good cells. We received even better results after round one than could have been expected.

The weeks in between sessions were awkward. Yes, I felt good. And yes, my prognosis was great. I also kept running, rode the bike a little, and remained in shape. But at the same time, this thing loomed over me and I didn't like it. I felt so good, I wanted to somehow expedite the process and press the fast forward button to get the next round of chemo behind me as well. As positive as I was trying to be,

I did have my darker moments. I didn't want to be perceived as sick and I didn't want to be sick.

Finally, round two was upon me. And it started with a bang. As promised, Monday of round two was to be a left-right combo punch of two drugs. The new drug being introduced, Rituxin was scheduled as a 4 hour infusion drip. Prior to that, I would also receive the Fludarabine that I had become accustomed to. I was relatively ok for the first 3 hours or so. But then had a pretty uncomfortable reaction to the Rituxin which included severe shakes and a fever of close to 102. The shakes were so bad, and the fever such a concern, that we stopped the treatment for about 20 minutes just so I could regroup. I remember telling my wife, MG, that I felt like I had been grinding up a tough hill in a race, and a race official just pulled me off the course and made me wait on the side of the road. I didn't feel like I was making any forward progress. I wasn't even walking my bike up the hill. For those brief few minutes, while the treatment was suspended, it felt like the cancer was winning.

But quickly enough, I was allowed to saddle up again, resume the race, and finish that day's stage. My nurse sent me home with two instructions. She wanted me to sleep in and not be the first one at the window the following day for treatment, and she didn't want me running when I got home. No worries on either count. My temp, body aches and shakes stayed with me through the night. I had experienced what Rituxin veterans refer to as "shake and bake syndrome". But finally, around midnight, the fever broke and I got some good rest. Remarkably, I was pretty much back to "normal" on Tuesday. Yes, I slept in a little. But given how bad I felt on Monday, I was amazed at how good I felt the very next day.

Tuesday's and Wednesday's treatments were pretty non eventful. I experienced no real side effects. I got in some light running, and even threw around some dumbbells for the hell of it. Thursday started out normal, but after treatment, my favorite nurse Mary Lou decided to draw some blood and send it to the lab. The results that came back were better than good. I had responded so well to the second round, that they were canceling chemo on Friday.

Now, while that sounds wonderful, the small print translation is that my WBCs and RBCs were getting pretty low - too low to blast them again with treatment. As expected, the chemo had taken out the good with the bad leaving me immune compromised and anemic. This result was going to happen anyway with sustained treatments; we just got there sooner than anticipated. So, instead of chemo on my last day of round two, I was given the WBC and RBC booster shots that were originally scheduled for the following week. I guess you could say I was ahead of schedule. I felt great, and I was even more optimistic. And I was very amazed at how positive the overall chemo experience was. I knew how lucky I was.

Blood would not be tested again for another week. During that time, I took extra precautions to avoid anything or anybody that might do damage to an already compromised immune system. I did however get in a few short runs and rides. In general, my spirits remained pretty high. They needed to be high to be able to fight the battle and to show everyone else I was ok and not suffering in bed with IV poles all around me. People would ask me how I felt in a soft and compassionate voice and I would snap back "GREAT!", "How are you?" At that, a few people looked perplexed and commented, "um, good … great …. Glad you feel so good". I wasn't being arrogant, just emphatic. I didn't want people putting me in their sick friend category. There were a couple of fleeting moments, where I would catch myself saying, "Holy crap, I have friggin cancer". But it was almost said in recognition of the irony of it all, and once recognized, I was able to move past it. It was like a check point for me to remember who the enemy was and then I would go on in good spirits.

Once I settled into a treatment routine, I don't think there was ever a time when I really felt vulnerable by this thing again. And if I did, the thought passed very quickly. The mystery had been removed. I knew what to expect with treatment and generally speaking I knew how I would likely respond. And as long as I was able to control what I could, I felt at ease with leaving the rest to the experts and the powers that be. So the goal at that point was to just maintain sanity, stay in shape, eat well, rest hard, and wait for the next doctor's appointment to gauge success and determine the next steps.

I headed back into chemo battle for round three on April 24th, 2006. I felt outstanding. I had an amazing 7 mile run the day before and I was really hard pressed to believe that I was sick. My blood work during that visit was completely normal. Seeing those results, and knowing how I felt, I decided to press my doctor a little bit. "Doc, you've examined me, you are happy with what you see. I feel outstanding. And my blood work is now normal. Is it safe for us to wrap the words partial remission around my condition at this point?" He paused briefly. And then turned away from his laptop and said, "No", you are not in partial remission, you are now in complete remission." I was so psyched that I wanted to run through the halls screaming. In exactly two months, I had reached the milestone that I was chasing. My wife and I just exchanged smiles that said it all. Suddenly, I settled back down and a thought then consumed me. I turned to him and asked, "Then why the hell am I going through another two rounds of this crap?"

Dr. Shore just smiled. "I knew that question was coming. Although you are in remission, history has told us that two rounds are not enough to do the complete job. We need to finish what we started and complete the full treatment protocol." He used the example of finishing a 10-day dose of an antibiotic even though you may feel better in a few days. He made sense. I was responding and recovering with minimal side effects. And I was really beginning to feel better, so I was content to carry on.

Round three also delivered really good news to me. Dr. Shore confirmed again that I was essentially out of the woods, and the remaining fourth round would be done simply to "finish my medicine". I was feeling better than I had felt in years. I was quickly realizing that my disease had been weighing me down for a while and I had no idea. And now I had no signs or symptoms at all of the disease. Even those pesky tonsils that started this ordeal had retreated back to normal size.

I realized that even though I had a round left, that round was academic and I had won. I hit remission within 60 days of diagnosis. My disease was now at a safe enough distance from me that I could go on with life and not worry about it, for the moment. And it left behind no ghost or reminder that would slow me down or make me alter my lifestyle in any way, for the moment. I could go full steam ahead. I felt faster and stronger than I had in years.

Emotionally, I felt completely healed. However intellectually, I understood this was a chronic form of leukemia with the potential to return at some point. But I wanted to celebrate my remission and focus on the here and now and not worry about what might happen down the road.

Speaking of That

By now you know the highlights and lowlights of my story... Healthy triathlon guy gets leukemia. Healthy triathlon guy gets treated and reaches remission. Healthy triathlon guy resumes racing. Healthy triathlon guy becomes a triathlon coach for Team in Training and an advocate for the disease. The end... err, no .... To be continued....

I have shared the details of that story and the many lives that have touched me, but I don't always share all of the details. There are some aspects to my story that I rarely mention. It's not that I am opposed to sharing, I just haven't. Maybe some parts are a little too personal, but every once in a while I will throw this out there into the universe. It's something that happened one night at home in between chemo cycles.

The Touch

In between rounds two and three of my initial treatments of chemo, something truly remarkable happened. Let me preface this by saying that my religion and spirituality has always been a personal thing with me. I was born, baptized and raised going to Presbyterian Church. I attended a Catholic college and studied a little world religion while there. I married into a Catholic family, in a Catholic church and picked up an interest in Eastern religions and philosophies along the way. My beliefs are Christian based with a commitment to doing what's right for the sake of what's right. Although admittedly, I'm not always certain where I fit.

So at the risk of sounding like I am preaching something, I will simply tell the story. I also need to add that there were many people who prayed very often and very hard for me, us, and my leukemia. All of their efforts are appreciated and I'm sure they all played a role in my positive outcome. However, there is one night that I feel is particularly worthy of mention. On April 12th, 2006 my wife's cousin Sharon and her husband John came to visit us.

The very brief background on Sharon is as follows: Sharon became very ill in the early 1990s with a condition that doctors simply could not get a handle on. She became bedridden, and wheelchair bound and was in excruciating pain. After many unsuccessful and futile conventional attempts with standard medical practices to try and diagnose and heal her, she finally turned to a healing prayer service. Immediately following one of these services, Sharon was on her feet and out of the chair. Within a week of attending this one particular service, Sharon was essentially cured and back to her normal self. Again, these are the facts; you arrive at your own conclusions.

Sharon and John came over to our house with the intention of praying for us and my disease. We spent some time getting caught up and hearing Sharon's amazing story and then Sharon and John settled down next to MG and I and started to pray over us. The first rather unusual or out of the ordinary thing we noticed was that our one dog immediately came over and started licking the hand of Sharon and vocalizing in a way that wasn't quite a bark, but more like a warning or that she wanted or sensed something. We had never seen or heard our dog behave like that in the past.

Shortly after that, Sharon placed her other hand on my forehead and continued to pray. This was "the touch" that did something to me. I immediately felt a combination of goose flesh and butterflies that originated in the pit of my stomach and radiated out to my extremities and through the top of my head. It seemed to last several minutes. And as this was happening my eyes suddenly began to tear up with no apparent advance emotion or warning. More like an involuntary direct response or reaction to something.

Shortly after that we ended our prayer. From that day on; I saw accelerated improvement in my condition. Certain lymph nodes which had been stubbornly enlarged and had not yet responded to chemo were reduced to normal size in 3 days. My next blood draw was considered normal even for normal people. And the round of chemo that I had after that yielded even better results than the first two had. By this time, my doctor had considered my condition in a state of full remission.

Draw your own conclusions… I drew mine immediately following "The Touch".

Oatmeal

Chemo brain is a very real thing. There are several textbook names for it. Names like chemotherapy induced cognitive dysfunction or cancer associated cognitive change, or post-chemotherapy cognitive impairment all describe the same thing. This happens during or after treatment and can have side effects that render the patient forgetful, unable to concentrate, unable to easily complete simple tasks, and generally just a few steps behind the world that may seem like it just picked up the pace.

From my personal experience, it usually happens after a few days of treatment and can resemble any or all of the following: That groggy feeling of being awakened from a sound sleep. Mild flu like symptoms with that feeling of a "full head". Feeling like you are submerged underwater and everything is a little cloudy and movement feels a little slower than what you would call normal.

Fret not. These are common symptoms associated with chemotherapy treatments. Specific symptoms and their severity will be different for everyone as no two people and their cancer experience will be identical. But the good news is, while there are exceptions to every rule, chemo brain typically doesn't last very long and just recognizing and indentifying the symptoms will help you relax and ride through them.

On another personal note, if I am going through a little bout of chemo brain I may not know if I want to take a shower, eat dinner, ride my bike, take a nap, cut the grass, or read a book. I just can't make decisions under those circumstances. So my loved ones and medical team have learned not to ask me what I want, but suggest a few options to limit the amount of thinking I need to do. But that's me.

Reasons

I am convinced that there are many "reasons" for my leukemia diagnosis just like there are reasons that have driven me to do the things that I have done as a result of my diagnosis. I may not always know what those reasons are, but the people that I have been able to connect with are too many to mention or even count. I wanted to take a minute and share just a couple of examples of people who have found me or stumbled upon me… or tripped over me as a result of my diagnosis. When I receive emails like the ones below, I feel like my disease has a greater sense purpose which gives me very clear direction.

Steve,

A friend of mine sent me the link to remissionman.com, and I felt the need to reach out to a fellow triathlete/former soccer player/leukemia surviving dad. After browsing your site, I'm beginning to think we're cosmically joined at the hip as the similarities are almost scary. I won't bore you with the details–you've lived them–but I just wanted to enlist you as a valuable member of my own support crew if you're willing. If there's one thing I've learned since I was diagnosed in late 2004, you can never have too many friends. Holler back if you get a moment. Until then, be well.

Steve,

It's great to read about your story. I was just starting triathlons before my surgery. Someday I'll get back to it. Gotta take care of a few things first... Keep up the good work!

Steve,

Thank you so much for your story. I too have CLL and am in complete remission. I am less fit and older and your story has inspired me to do something about the "fit" part. Thanks again. Good luck.

Steve,

You are a true inspiration. I am Vince's wife Janet and I relived your struggles. Vince and you are very similar. Janet Papale

Steve,

My husband came upon the feature article on you in the January issue of Endurance NEWS. While CLL is probably more common than people realize, we have never seen any articles written about people, athletes like you, who have had this disease.

I was diagnosed with CLL in 1996 at the age of 47 because of blood work that I had requested just for a good physical only to find my white count was higher than normal. The doctors just kept an eye on it but it never subsided and in 2000 I began therapy and had an autologous bone marrow transplant. I was out of remission after 5 years and again we played the wait and see game. I will be starting chemo in March to try and get back into remission.

I have been biking for many years as well as skiing, doing some weight training and anything else to keep healthy. I think I have succeeded with as much as I am able to control. I have always felt good except during treatment.

I guess the point of writing to you is to try to find out as much as I can about what you did to keep yourself fit-Hammer products in particular as well as your nutrition in general. I am very active and do follow a good diet-except for the love of chocolate, dark of course.

The article actually was refreshing compared to all of the depressing articles on the internet which I have stopped reading long ago. I want to remain as active and as vibrant as possible not only for myself but for my husband and 6 grandchildren. I really don't have time for set backs. Please let me know what you did, what your treatments consisted of, and how your disease progressed.

Steve,

I read your bio on your web site and was very intrigued. I guess I am sending this email because I too have a story. 1 1/2 years ago I quit smoking and drinking and began running. I did my first sprint triathlon (Irongirl) last August and have completed 2 marathons so far. Not only that but in 1995 I was diagnosed with Multiple Sclerosis. I just became a certified fitness trainer as well. I too want to be people's inspiration. I believe if I could do these things anyone can. I want to help people have their own stories to inspire others; I am not sure how to do this, any advice?

Hi Steve,

Not sure if you remember me or not. My wife was recently diagnosed with cancer I am looking for more info. I see you do a lot with local groups and more. If you could pass along any info I would appreciate it. I'm possibly looking into walks or runs, or just anything.

Some Days

While I don't dwell on this fact, a day doesn't go by where I am not aware of the fact that I have leukemia. I may feel perfectly healthy with no signs or symptoms of the disease, yet… I still know it lives inside me. It's not something that I put on or take off, but it's something that I always wear. Generally speaking, I'm OK with that because I know I have it in a good place and I know I manage my disease very well. I've said before that I look at my disease as something I've been given to see what I can turn it into.

Perhaps chronic lymphocytic leukemia needed a voice or a poster child. So why not choose me? My footprint is pretty large and I usually have a pretty good outlook on most things. So I get it. I understand why I was chosen to carry this thing around with me. But now that it's been 9 years since my diagnosis, I feel like it might be nice to give this thing a day off once in a while.

While I am so fortunate to have people that care about me the way they do, I am only human. I have my moments and even my days and weeks. Some days it gets tiring hearing people ask the question. It's a question that seems innocent and harmless to most people but to someone living with a disease, it takes on a whole new meaning. When someone asks "How are you feeling?" It conjures up a lot of the dark thoughts that are sometimes associated with something like this. I'm often quick to snap back that I feel "FINE!" And almost resent them asking in the first place.

For me, that one simple question triggers a lot more dialogue inside my own head… "Why, don't I look ok?" "Why, do you know something that I don't?" "Why are you obsessing over my disease?" And at times I want to just blurt out that I'm perfect and to drop the subject. But I know better. I genuinely appreciate that people care enough about me to ask. I know they mean well and truly care. I've learned over time to give them just enough of a response to satisfy their sincere inquiry. Enough that says "Check up was great, blood work was great, and I feel great." Then I change the subject and move on.

Some days this thing gets old. But I guess that's the beauty of tomorrow.

Leukemia Lessons Learned

The top 10 lessons I have learned during my initial diagnosis and subsequent treatments of my leukemia.

Blood cancers do not play by any rules.

Stuff can happen to anybody.

"Stuff" doesn't measure our character, how we react and respond to that "stuff" does.

The internet is full of as much useless information as useful. Talk to doctors and choose your websites and content wisely. Don't just blindly search a disease.

A strong mind and will are amazing forces and should not be underestimated.

Support crews are critical.

Chemotherapy nurses are among the most special people on the planet.

Don't be afraid to ask questions and get second and third opinions.

Eating elephants is easiest one bite at a time.

Some incredibly positive things can be done with what might initially seem like very negative news.

Be Where Your Feet Are

Earlier this year, I had an opportunity to talk to athletes from Cabrini College. That was fun for me as I graduated from Cabrini many lifetimes ago so I enjoy visiting the campus whenever I can. I went in totally cold and unscripted so I wasn't sure how I was going to frame whatever I was going to say. I knew the group would be small and it would give me an opportunity to fully engage them for who they are and just let the talk have its own set of legs and lungs and go wherever it needed to. A few interesting questions were asked and I could tell that most of the room seemed pretty dialed into what I was saying. I think I touched on a few things that resonated with them.

I talked about a lot of things ranging from family life to Cabrini life to triathlon life, and of course life with leukemia. A few of the key points that I honed in on were around the choices we make and our reactions and responses to the cards that we are dealt. And some of you have heard me talk about this many times. Sometimes we get so stuck in the muck complaining about what happened TO us that we neglect opportunities to respond in a positive light and take some of that control back and do something FOR ourselves.

I reminded the group to think about the size of their footprints and not the sound of their footsteps. One doesn't need to display a large billboard to show the world your accomplishments. When you do things right, people will just know. Your accomplishment becomes you without needing to draw attention to it – or yourself. I've always thought there is grace and class in accomplishing huge feats with quiet subtlety.

I also talked about my passion for coaching the Team in Training triathlon crew. I encouraged them to find something in this world that they love, and look for ways to use it in a way that might also benefit others.

One student athlete asked me how I stay mentally focused in a long race or training day. Admittedly, that's hard to do. And I have certainly done my share of unraveling from time to time. But my response to him pulled from a quote that a friend shared with me. This friend was a long time professional soccer goalkeeper with a brilliant career that took him all over the world. He once told me that he is now happy just enjoying life's simple pleasures and doing regular yoga. He told me time has taught him the importance of "being where your feet are". I think about that often if I let things get too far ahead of me and feel overwhelmed. I focus on staying in the moment and simply remind myself to be where my feet are.

One of the last questions of the night came from the assistant swim coach. He wanted to know how I want to be remembered decades from now. The timing of this question was eerie because the night before, I received a very nice note from an old college friend that pretty much answered the question. This friend had stumbled onto my website and told me that she loved my blog and reminded me of a day many many years ago that she blew out her knee in a friendly game of "touch" football at Cabrini. I borrowed a car, took her to the hospital, stayed with her and made sure she was taken care of. She also told me that I officially nicknamed her "wheels" from that day forward.

She went on to say how much she appreciated what I did and let me know she has never forgotten that day. She also said "you were giving then, and I see you still are". And that my friends, is how I would like to be remembered. I think if you give of yourself and expect nothing in return, and you don't take yourself too seriously, then you have discovered the secret of happiness.

Connections

I want to share the story of another important connection that I made during this trek. I received the below email from a woman whose father was just recently diagnosed with the same form of leukemia that I was diagnosed with. Needless to say, I was very touched by her email. So much so, that I made arrangements to meet the woman, as well as her mom, during the weekend of the Philadelphia Marathon. We met briefly after the race and established a great connection which I hope will continue to grow.

Read on ...

I am a 22 year old recent Penn graduate and now a nurse at HUP in Philadelphia. I was reading over the Philly Magazine Be Well Blog and came across your name and story. I just wanted to tell you that you are an inspiration for me. My family found out in May that my 49 year old father (who has never been sick in his life) was diagnosed with CLL. While he does not have any symptoms and is lucky to be Stage 0 at this time, this sudden diagnosis was shocking and devastating to us, especially since it is not common for people so young to be diagnosed with CLL.

My father has always been my hero and the person I aspire to be like, which sounds cliché but is 100% true. Since my mother and I are both nurses, we knew the seriousness of this diagnosis and my mother especially has been having a really hard time trying to come to terms with my father's diagnosis. She has talked to many people who know someone who received the same diagnosis and she tends to focus on the worst-case scenarios. Reading about your story made me so excited to show her an example of someone who was diagnosed young, just like my father, and who has pushed through and fought this illness into remission. While we have no idea what is in store for my father and his fight with CLL, it's always nice to hear of a good outcome.

I don't want to take up a lot of your time, but I saw you are running in this Saturday's 8k run. I took up running myself just before we received my father's diagnosis and it has helped give me an outlet to escape the worry that is sometimes prevalent in my family and explore what my body is capable of. My father's diagnosis encouraged me to sign up for this race and I can't believe it is finally here. I just wanted to let you know that I am even more excited to cross the finish line this Saturday knowing you are running in this race as well and I hope you know how much of an inspiration you are to people like me.

If you happen to see a girl with black pants and a red long sleeved Penn shirt on amongst the hundreds of people on Saturday, please say hello. My mom will be there to cheer me on and I can't wait to send this e-mail and tell her about your story. Thank you so much for your story and good luck Saturday!

A Few More Questions

As you will hear me say many times over, my multisport and cancer networks have become huge as a result of how public I have been with my story. I love when people just find me as they are out there in cyber space researching their disease, or sport, or both. My athlete / patient profile was recently featured on the website workoutcancer.org whose mission is to support **pilot and pre-clinical studies investigating the effects of exercise on physiology and on cancer treatments. Pretty interesting stuff. I loved how concise the questions were and thought they were worthy of sharing. Below are my responses to a few of their questions.**

When was your diagnosis and how did you find out you had cancer?
February 24th, 2006. In the preceding couple of months, I was having some difficulty swallowing. At first it was

solid foods but the difficulty progressed to simply swallowing saliva. A consult with an ear, nose, and throat specialist revealed enlarged tonsils so a tonsillectomy was ordered. Pre admission blood work testing revealed an elevated white count and I was referred to an oncologist. Additional blood work, a CT scan, PET scan, x-rays, and a bone marrow biopsy all clearly indicated chronic lymphocytic leukemia.

What was your treatment plan and how far after treatment are you?

The initial plan called for four one-week cycles. Treatment ran one week on, followed by three weeks off. The drugs used were Fludara and Rituxan. After that, I required follow up maintenance treatment with just Rituxan every six months for two years. I have since "relapsed" twice; once in 2012 and once in 2013. My relapses were quickly tamed with a combination of the steroid Decadron and additional Rituxan.

How physically active were you before diagnosis?

Extremely. I have been an athlete my entire life. I played semi professional soccer for a number of years and started racing in the mid 1980s. By the time I was diagnosed, I was already a veteran ironman triathlete and marathon runner.

How did your physical activity change, if at all, prior to, during, and after treatment?

After a long heart to heart discussion with my doctor, he agreed to allow me to remain as active as possible during my treatments, with the caveat that I would listen to my body when it told me to rest. When I felt good, I often ran home from chemo. And I worked especially hard during my three weeks off in between cycles to rebuild my strength. I was back to racing a few months after my initial treatments and raced an iron distance triathlon seven months post diagnosis.

Regarding your cancer experience and physical activity, what benefits/drawbacks did you notice?

I really feel that remaining active (and already being in good shape) was a catalyst in helping me reach remission quickly. There were a few times that I really needed to dial everything back down and do nothing but rest. But I understood that to be cyclical and after rest, I would be able to bounce back again.

What physical activity milestones have you had throughout your cancer survivorship experience?

The one that stands out the most is the iron distance triathlon I did seven months post diagnosis. The race director was one of my "go to" people throughout my treatment journey. He was a mentor, a friend, and an expert in the medical field. He renamed me "RemissionMan" when I crossed that finish line and told a heart warming rendition of the story at the race's awards brunch.

Regarding cancer treatment(s), what advice would you offer newly diagnosed cancer patients about physical activity and quality of life?
Be patient. This process is full of peaks and valleys, which is very much like endurance racing. Take things one day, one treatment, and one mile at a time.

Anything else that you would like to mention?
Stay the course. You are NOT in this fight alone.

Maintaining & Monitoring

After my initial remission in 2006 I settled in to a regular routine of follow up appointments with my doctor. I would see him every 3-6 months to check my blood counts and chat about how I was feeling. For the most part that became an uneventful exercise. Although I did and still do get a little anxious in the days leading up to my appointments. Even if I thought I was feeling fine I knew the true gauge of my disease related health was my blood results. There were other red flags to be monitored and taken into consideration when determining my status, but those blood levels were most important to me. If I got a clean bill, then Mary Grace and I would do our signature happy dance leaving the office and I could go on with my life worry free until the next appointment.

The one real annoyance with this disease is the need to check in with my doctor with things that I normally would not see a doctor for. For example, I was never one to run to the doc with coughs or congestion, but he wanted me to check in with him any time I was feeling under the weather. I've learned to respect and understand this a little more over time. Having a slightly compromised immune system, I really needed to keep things like this in check. Plus you never know what might mark the return of something more that just a cough.

When it was time for my semi annual Rituxin maintenance treatments, I felt like an old veteran of the chemo suite. I knew that battlefield like the back of my hand and I had become accustomed to seeing some of the same nurses and patients. The routine was pretty consistent. Every six months for two years I would report in for a five day dose of my favorite monoclonal antibody. I had the option of taking this every day for five days, or spreading it out over five consecutive Mondays. I opted for the latter. This also let me continue to work a condensed week around my treatments.

I developed a love - hate relationship with Rituxan. This drug worked for me. I got great results where some folks cannot even tolerate it. For that I feel very fortunate. But the flip side is that I often teetered on the border of having certain reactions to it. If they administered this too quickly, I would react with a fever, hives, sweats, etc. But as long as the drip rate was slowed down to an intermittent trickle, I seemed to tolerate it. I also seemed to tolerate it better over time and with subsequent treatments. We all had an understanding that when Steve Brown checked in for day one of Rituxan treatment, it was going to be a very long day. This stuff is a little bit like working with dynamite. It blows stuff up really well, but you really don't want to get too close to it.

It probably goes against every preconceived notion you may have to say that my chemo experiences were positive, but they were. I was surrounded by positive people who were taking very good care of me. I had plenty of food, drink, and reading or listening material to keep me satisfied and occupied. Mary Grace sat by my side all day, and my kids sometimes popped in to hang out with us as well. The chemo suite is not a dark and dungeon like toxin chamber filled with sick people. It's a place of healing and hope filled with incredibly positive people.

Throughout all of this, I continued to strengthen and grow the relationship I had formed with Team in Training. Since 2006 we recruited and trained athletes for two to three different triathlons each year. Every athlete had a story and a reason for being part of the team. Coaching them and watching them grow and develop and then seeing their faces as they crossed the finish line is like hitting the lottery for me. My involvement with that organization brought everything full circle and was just further justification for having this disease.

I also maintained my own schedule of racing and training which took me to some amazing places, and connected me with some amazing people. Longer races such as ironman triathlons and marathons often hinged on clean check ups from my oncologist. Which was great for me because it gave me added confidence that I really was ok and had the green light to push the limits.

Our Toes Aren't Always in the Sand

A friend recently reached out to me looking for advice for herself and for her friend who was recently diagnosed with a terminal illness. I thought I would share some of my response.

This is a tough one and I'm really sorry for everyone dealing with this. There are a number of things that I did that helped me both process what I was going though, and help with some of the physical and emotional side effects. These may or may not work for someone else but hopefully she can take at least one thing away from my experiences.

One thing that helped me dramatically was to write about my experiences. This doesn't need to be anything formal and can be anything from a blog to an email to yourself, or just a running journal of thoughts and feelings. This helped me identify and process a lot of what I was going though.

Also, music was key for me. While I can't play a single lick of anything on any instrument, I am a music junkie. So just being able to get lost in my music was another way to escape and relax my mind. In many cases the music and the writing went hand in hand.

I don't know what her level of energy is or will be but of course activity was really important for me as well. If she is up for it and can get out to walk, it may help. It paid huge dividends for me.

Her support team is in a tough spot because you all want to do the right thing by her but sometimes you don't know what that is. Hell, she may not even know what she wants or what she needs. And if she does articulate those needs, they may and probably will change and change often. Couple all of that with your own sadness and it can be a tough thing to manage. So one of the best pieces of advice that I can give you is to ask her what you can do or be for her. Give her control and ask her to direct you guys. You are her team. If you walk timidly around her and her situation, she will do the same. If you open the door to talk about her feelings and fears openly, she will follow that lead as well.

She may want to walk. She may want to talk. She may want to write or listen to music. She may want to look through pictures and relive some of those memories. Or she may want to cry. Ask her what she wants to do right now in this moment. And also, when the time is right, ask her what you all can do in her name and in her honor. But for now, be alive with her and embrace every exchange.

Happy to continue this conversation with you and whoever.

First Relapse

Living with a chronic disease like chronic lymphocytic leukemia is like living with a caged up wild cat in your basement. You do your best to keep it locked and chained and barricaded away. You live your life with an "out of sight, out of mind" mentality. Intellectually, you need to be aware that you have a huge and sometimes angry cat locked away in a room downstairs, but emotionally, you can't let it own you. So you work hard at holding those reminders at a safe distance. You work hard at doing the right things and address those things requiring attention, and turn blinders to the rest.

In 2012 I was starting to have a few uncomfortable symptoms that very much resembled what I felt when I was first diagnosed. I checked in with my oncologist and did the normal blood workup along with a CT scan. And as suspected, a few CLL symptoms had returned. This was its first official curtain call since my original diagnosis. The CT scan showed very pronounced lymph nodes in my neck and in my throat. We talked about a number of potential treatment options and next steps. My symptoms were very localized and while my tonsils and lymph nodes were impacted, the rest of my body was still rather "normal" as was my blood work. So that ruled out a conventional chemo or monoclonal antibody treatment but we wanted to do something which would knock this thing back off the radar again.

We agreed on an aggressive four day round of the high dosage mega steroid Decadron and gauged the results along the way. This is a relatively standard quasi treatment option in cases like this when some symptoms are present but not enough to warrant full blown chemo. Now, I mentioned having a love - hate relationship with Rituxan. I can't say the same about Decadron. I don't have an ounce of love in me for Decadron. It's true that it is a powerful steroid and works well, but the downside is that this stuff winds me up pretty tightly and I don't sleep – at all. But I agreed that this was a logical next step and we could always change direction if need be.

While I can't say that my Decadron treatments were enjoyable, I can say they were effective. I had many sleepless nights which spilled into long days which turned into bouts of anxiety and even depression. But the stuff worked in that I was free of any signs or symptoms of the leukemia. All the while, life had to carry on. Work had to carry on. And my passions for coaching, training, and racing obviously carried on. When I could, I scheduled the treatments around whatever else was happening on the calendar (Including Ironman Eagleman 70.3 that June).

It's true that the Decadron treatments worked but the trade offs were difficult to manage and as it turned out, the results didn't last for long. A short couple of months after my Decadron treatments, symptoms returned. The solution this time was pretty simple. Given the fact that I had a good track record with Rituxan, the call was made for six rounds of "smart bomb" therapy administered once per week. I tolerated everything this time like an old pro and my response was excellent. Given my history, we again started out very slowly but were able to increase the drip rate along the way.

My daughter Jennifer and her wife Lauren joined my for treatment number two. While drifting in and out of a nap in the chair, I received a text message from my good friend and fellow cancer warrior Ethan Zohn. He knew where I was because we chatted earlier in the day. Ethan asked the million dollar question "Are you running home?" I did the responsible thing and waited until I was completely finished treatment to even think about the answer to that question. But I felt so good when I was done; I had to make that run. Jennifer joined me on that run home. It was extremely cool on many levels.

For me, running home post chemo is one of the most rewarding and gratifying things I can possibly do to regain control. I sometimes feel a little helpless (and bored) sitting in a chemo chair for hours on end. But when I am unleashed, and feel good enough to run home, all of the momentum and positive energy shifts back into my corner. It feels like I regain complete control of my disease, my life, and everything in it. I celebrate the run, and trash talk the leukemia.

Things went so well that by treatment number three they were able to rapidly infuse me and I was out of there in 90 minutes. Of course Mary Grace was with me and we celebrated that session perhaps even more so than any other. When we checked in on the morning of my fourth treatment we were greeted with a wonderful surprise. My doctor walked in the room and after having reviewed my blood work he asked when I wanted to come back and see him again. Of course my wife and I looked at him a little strange and said, "Next week I suppose…just like I've been doing for the last four weeks. Today is only number four of six so I still have two more to go after today." In response to that came these magical words: "Oh, no, sorry. I only want you to do four treatments in total. I would have only stretched to six if I was worried about anything and I needed to keep that option open. But I'm worried not at all. We've accomplished what we needed to accomplish and you are officially back in remission so you are done after today." That was a wonderful present to receive on Mary Grace's birthday.

It was pouring down rain when we left, so I decided not to run home from treatment that day. But, I did hop on the indoor trainer and do some riding to give this disease a few more kicks to the head, for good measure. Because I could.

Life's Ring of Keys

With each passing day I am reminded more and more how all of this stuff is connected and how each of us are somehow related to our neighbor. And with each passing day, I am reminded that the lessons I've learned about life, about dealing with disease, about work, about sports, or about anything else you can name, all boil down to a handful of common denominators that when realized provide a sense of acceptance, clarity, and comfort.

For starters, we need to understand that we are all writing our autobiographies with everything we do each and every day. So what are we choosing to write? A bestselling thriller? Or a mediocre story that will quickly end up in the back of the discount rack? We own it. It's ours. We are our own writer, producer, director, cameraman, editor, lead actor, and for that matter – critic. So let's write our story the way we want to be remembered.

All too often people are paralyzed and motionless like a deer in headlights afraid to take that first step simply because they can't see the entire staircase in front of them. Do we really have to care or worry? What's important is that the staircase is sound and that you are sure-footed as you go. You don't need the full road map right now this minute to be able to make your next move. Follow your heart and follow your instincts.

We all have bad days. The truth is we all have some REALLY bad days. Hopefully we have many more good than bad. But whatever is making up your bad day, there is one universal truth. The sun will set on that bad day. And as has been the case for every one of my days so far in my lifetime, a new day will be here tomorrow. With healthy perspective and a little luck, that day should bring a renewed sense of hope and possibility. Good or bad, most of the emotions that we experience in life will be cyclical. The secret is to remember that and dress accordingly to ride out the storm while always remembering to cherish the good times, no matter how long they may last. Another one will return.

We have far more choices than we sometimes care to admit. It's sometimes easier to play the victim card and not take action because of something that has happened to us. While we don't always have control over those happenings, we have full control over how we react and how we respond. Choose wisely.

It's ok to kick and scream and find fault when things don't go as we hope they would; but only very briefly. Very soon you will need to pick yourself up and either resume your journey or chart a new course. And how do you do that? By not fearing the first step even if you can't see that whole staircase.

Have the courage to do the right thing even if it's not the most popular thing.

Did you ever notice there are certain people who brighten a room just by walking through the door? They possess a certain intangible quality that attracts goodness and light. They may not even have to say a word. They may just "be". Figure out what those qualities are and choose to be one of those people.

You can't have enough friends, allies, and loved ones. But you should make it a point to let the people who are important to you, know that they matter. And it's never too late to make that acknowledgement. I still reach out to teachers I had decades ago just to say thanks.

Things aren't always fair. Accept that and move on. But always try to create a level playing field and one of complete acceptance for everyone in your world, even if you may have been dealt a rough hand. Turn it around and make it count for something positive for someone else. Be a facilitator of positive change.

Play is good for the body, mind, and soul. Do it more often.

Laughter is good for the body, mind, and soul. Do it more often.

Surround yourself with people who respect who you are on good days and bad. A little objective disagreeing is healthy and provides balance, but never sacrifice integrity and respect in yourself or in those you choose to spend time with.

This is really a pretty simple thing. I'm not sure why we choose to complicate matters.

Giving Thanks

This is the time of year that I , like many others, take a few inventories and remind myself of all of the things that matter, and that I am grateful for. The important thing for me to remember is that things always have a way of working their way out. The "downs" seem to always rebound and at the end of the day, I am still ahead of the game. So let's take a few minutes and appreciate all that we have.

Be thankful for your leaky roof because at least you have one over your head.

Be thankful for the boss you may dislike for you must be employed.

Be thankful that you finished dead last in a recent race because you had the courage to start.

Be thankful that while disease sucks, we live in a time of incredible technology and advancement.

Be thankful for everyone in your family because you are blessed to have one.

Be thankful for how fortunate you are to be able to complain to a food server about your meal.

Be thankful for your broken heart. It means you know how to love, and will love again.

Be thankful for the guy who cuts you off in traffic since you could be walking.

Be thankful for all of the snow you will shovel… from your own driveway and walk…. In front of your own home.

Be thankful that you are blessed with the freedom of choice in this world.

Too Many Too Few

Below are a few words that I sent to a good friend as he prepared for another round of battle by way of a stem cell transplant. Although it was written for Ethan Zohn, it can easily serve as a battle cry for anyone going through their own situation. Our team is a united team.

Many too many play the "why me" card when it comes to things like cancer. They take the easy route and give in to the disease and all of the evil that goes with it.
Many too many focus on what they don't have and how much they hurt. They worry in vain about the hair or weight that they've lost.
Many too many are anchors in their own healing process and have no idea how much control they really have

Too few are those like you who can mentally, spiritually, and emotionally rise above it. They have the gift of being able to sift through the dirt until they find that ray of hope. Too few are those like you who can let that ray of hope guide them. They lead by example and spread their message of possibility for all to see.

Too few are those like you with the courage to allow themselves to be truly seen. They may have patches of physical weakness but never do they really feel beaten

Just know that although this war may seem long, you are winning.

Just understand that the team in your fox hole is larger than your wildest dreams.

Just realize that you are helping countless people in their own struggles just by being.

Just believe that this will soon be a speed bump in your rear view mirror.

Just keep the perspective and the faith.

Just use this as a chance to continue to make a difference in this world.

Building the Perfect Beast

The spark that ignited this post is the 1984 album of the same name by former Eagle Don Henley. I have always been intrigued by the title and often find myself using it when I talk about putting the pieces of something together. Particularly in multisport training as athletes are constantly trying to strike the perfect balance of several critical components such as training volume, rest, nutrition, equipment, family, work, etc. The goal of every athlete is to try to put all of the pieces together that will yield the best result. And with proper planning & preparation, a little luck and perhaps some divine intervention, hopefully you will have built a (near) perfect beast come race day.

But the title speaks to much more than multisport training. "The Beast" concept hit me again the other day when I was responding to a friend's email and I realized that I am constantly in a state of building or creating something or charting a course to somewhere. And I'm not positive I yet know what it is that I am building or where it is that I am going. I'm still not 100% certain of some of my "reasons" for the people that I meet and often don't know what lies ahead but I feel as though I am frequently being guided in one direction or another for a particular reason. And that typically leads me to something or someone who seems to be able to provide the next building block or the next direction to turn on my path.

To view things in an even bigger perspective, building the "Beast" is our perpetual mission to connect everything in this world until we have a fully united and integrated yet diversified entity and platform with which to do great things. No more silos, no more individualized agendas. Just one giant glowing sphere of brotherly awesome… the Perfect Beast.

Years ago I was a soccer goalkeeper and one of the professional athletes that I admired was a guy named Shep Messing. Well somehow we connected a few years ago and have remained in touch. And it was Shep who introduced me to another goalkeeper – Ethan Zohn, who had just been diagnosed with lymphoma. Shep did his part in building the beast because he sensed a connection would be valuable for Ethan and I. And he was right.

It happened again not too long ago when I received the following email from a friend:

Hi Steve,
I have a 26 year old young lady who would like to donate volunteer time to work with people who are struggling with cancer. She is in her last semester of college finishing a degree in counseling. I have been working with her and can attest to her character and nature. I would greatly appreciate it if you can help us connect her with the right people/agency to be of service.
Thanks In Advance

Ironically, the above email came from another former soccer goalkeeper who now works with kids in a local school district and is giving back and paying it forward in very big ways. In my playing days, obviously I had no idea how significant the goalie connection would become. Although I always did recognize goalies as being a special breed…. with unique camaraderie.

Of course I will be able to connect the woman referenced in the email. And who knows how many lives she may end up touching, or saving. And how many lives those people may touch. It's all part of an ever evolving process. Someday perhaps I will be able to look back on all of this and fully understand how all of the jig saw pieces have fit together. Until that day, I remain very happy to be able to fit pieces in here and there and connect smaller chunks of the puzzle. And I feel very fortunate for the things I have done, the places I have seen, and the people I have met. I know that it is all leading to something very good and very positive; I just can't quite make out the full picture just yet. Things are still incomplete and fuzzy. But that's all ok.

And keeping within the music theme, I think I find myself "On the Road to Find Out" as Cat Stevens once wrote. And I'm good with that. I'm fine with not knowing all of the answers because I am doing exactly what I remind others to do all of the time. And that is I am enjoying the journey. Don't fret too much about the destination or how fast you get there. But keep your eyes, ears, and heart open so that you can process and enjoy everything along the way. Happiness is a journey and not a destination.

Keeping Demons at Your Back

By now you probably all too familiar with my story. But I need to reiterate a couple of things. I have always been a fitness junkie so I was a little unsure how treatments would impact my lifestyle – which could have had a pretty negative impact on me emotionally. Luckily, my doctor and I reached an agreement and he allowed me to continue to train through and in between treatments as long as I felt good. When I was tired, I promised I would rest. But when I felt good – I worked out.

Since I was treated as an out patient, I often ran back home after my chemo treatments. Part of it was to try to control SOMETHING in a relatively uncontrollable situation. Part of it was just to try to stay fit. But part of it was also to send a message to the cancer that I was not going to lie around the house and be a victim. This ended up being a very empowering move which I am sure aided my swift remission.

Granted not everyone is a runner, but simply walking and moving or doing something during an illness and treatment can help keep you balanced and focused. And that sense of emotional well being and stability has to have a positive effect on your overall healing process.

Get out and move. Enjoy the moment, the day, and the scenery, whatever. Just do yourself a favor and get active. It is one of the most effective methods of therapy around! And it's FREE.

Relapse Take Two

2013 again saw the return of some problematic and enlarged lymph nodes. My blood work showed an elevated white count with a higher concentration of lymphocyte cells. A CT scan revealed that the majority of my lymph nodes were again enlarged and on the move. Nodes in my neck, chest, armpit, groin, etc. were all showing signs of growth. And of course my tonsils, which were always the biggest red flag, were larger again. So we opted to go through some additional treatment and the hope was I could work these in and around a couple of remaining races I had on my calendar.

This time we used the same drug we had previous success with – Rituxan. The game plan called for a slighter higher dosage to be administered once per month over three to four months depending on how the results looked along the way. Accompanying the Rituxan was the steroid and my familiar foe Decadron.

My initial round started off ok but about an hour in, I started to have somewhat of an allergic reaction around my neck. As the nurses evaluated this, we hypothesized that the probable cause for the reaction was actually a very cool one. Rituxan has smart bomb characteristics and knows to zero in on inflamed lymphatic organs only. Given the high concentration of enlarged lymph nodes in my neck, it made sense that this reaction was merely the Rituxan kicking the crud out of the enlarged lymph nodes but causing a reaction as it did. I could actually feel the effects of the drug the way you could envision peroxide working on an open cut or wound. I thought that was a pretty awesome concept to think about. Even so, we were forced to halt the treatment for a few minutes to give me a chance to normalize. Once we started back up at a slower drip rate and I took a little more Benadryl, I seemed to be OK.

Later in the afternoon I developed a little nausea but that too subsided after an additional dose of Compazine. My day ended around 3:30 PM. It was a little long, but not that bad. As usual, my favorite nurse Mary Lou was all over my every want and need and took excellent care of me. And of course Mary Grace was with me every step of the way, bringing me coffee, lunch, and Swedish Fish. And thanks too to our daughter Danielle who also visited and brought in some treats, and a Sponge Bob Square Pants balloon. Plenty of love and positive energy also came from our crew in Yuma Arizona. While they may be across the country, they are always front and center in our hearts. I felt pretty normal the next day and was able to get back to work and plan for the NYC Marathon which I was scheduled to run in between sessions.

I was met with some additional challenges over the next couple of treatments. All of them were adverse reactions to the Rituxan. Again, I love it because it's effective, but it's a bitch to live with at times. The next session started out as most of them do. MG and I had breakfast in the hospital cafeteria then made our way up to Dr. Shore's office before heading back down to the chemo suite. My blood work was good with no issues to report at all. So after we reiterated "the plan" and talked about dosing and timing, etc., MG and I did the traditional "my blood work is normal" happy dance in the hallway.

My favorite chemo nurse met us, ushered us in, and got me all set up. I started out pretty smoothly. My musical taste was just as scattered as usual and I jumped around between an old 1973 Lindsay Buckingham and Stevie Nicks album, to Peter Gabriel's Secret World Tour, to Yes Fragile, to Of Monsters and Men, to The Postal Service, to Dave Matthews, to Lorde, to Cat Stevens. I drifted on and off in the recliner for a few minutes at a time. My attention tends to dart around the room and from TV to iPad to phone like a repeating loop. I'm usually interrupted by regular vital sign checks and by the fact that I have to constantly pee with all of the fluids being pumped into me. So my pole and I have to get up and take frequent walks to the rest room for excitement. Of course MG brought me my lunch and sat with me while getting caught up on some work of her own.

The issue I had this time was another hive-like allergic reaction to the Rituxan. So we needed to stop for a few minutes, push a little extra Benadryl through my IV and wait for me to settle down. I did settle down and the added Benadryl must have knocked me out a little because the remainder of that IV bag seemed to empty pretty fast. I was surprised that after four and a half hours I was done "already". As Mary Lou was unhooking me and bandaging me up, I tried to look out the window to see what the weather was doing. It looked clear and that gave me the brilliant idea of wanting to run home. I knew I felt good enough to do it. MG was a little hesitant for all of the right reasons but we both knew it would be good for me. MG didn't think Mary Lou would approve however. But I knew that Mary Lou wouldn't have a care in the world, because I sure as hell wasn't going to tell her.

We made our way to MG's car; I dropped off my stuff, gave her a kiss, and made my way out of the garage and began my run. (I think it was easier running than navigating the after school traffic in a vehicle). MG asked which way I would be going just in case she needed to loop back and look for me. I chose the longer of the two routes home for a few reasons. None of them are that important. About 5 minutes later I heard the familiar honk of our Chevy Equinox and I just smiled and threw both arms triumphantly in the air. As she drove past and waved, I smiled and said to myself...

"Yep"

I finished my remaining treatment without any major issues and settled back in to a safe and comfortable place affectionately referred to as remission. The Decadron did make it a little difficult to sleep, but the Benadryl helped offset that little bit. At times it feels like all I do is take something to offset something else. This is a chronic form of leukemia that I live with. There may be times that symptoms may reappear, when they do, we zap them off the radar. I respond well to the treatments. And all things considered, this poses very little inconvenience to me or my lifestyle. I'm confident that with drug advancements the way they are, my magic vitamin is right around the corner which will radically change current treatment protocols.

At the end of the day, our sanity and happiness comes down to three things. 1). Understanding that much of what we go through in this life will be cyclical but we should work really hard to remain where our feet are. 2) Understanding that we have control over many of our choices. 3). Being able to accept and effectively manage the "Plan B" when we have to.

Remission ROCKS.

Words You Long to Hear (and say)

I wanted to share one small blurb of an email that I received from a friend who was recently diagnosed. These are words that every patient lives to be able to say. And everyone else prays to be able to hear:

"As for me, I am on the upswing from the transplant. My new cells engrafted very quickly which was great. I am still fighting off some of the other side effects that follow a BMT, but am hoping for discharge to home sometime next week. Can't wait to get out of here!"

A Matter of Perspective

Perspective; I use that word all the time. It's all about perspective…it depends on your perspective …keep it all in perspective. Singer songwriter John Gorka has a great song about being a native of New Jersey. He sings about the girls with the high hair and measuring your socio economic status in terms of Jersey Turnpike exits. In the song he also says "If the world were to end tomorrow, I would adjust". How's that for adaptability and perspective? Maybe John Gorka is a triathlete. Or a cancer survivor.

At any rate, I often find myself keeping or putting things into perspective. A few key concepts help keep my perspective on track. First point … things are rarely as bad as they first appear. I always try to remember that there are many people who are far less fortunate than I. I have a roof over my head, an amazing family, a great network of friends, my health, and I am gainfully employed in the best nation in the world. For all intents and purposes, my life is a fairy tale.

I also try to remember that most issues and problems are typically short term in the grand scheme of things. In most cases, there will be an end. So, the bigger challenge is not in the crises itself, but in how we accept and manage the crises. That is what will drive our degree of happiness. And that is a choice that we all have. We choose to be happy or not by how we relate to what goes on around us. And how do we do that? We do so by keeping things in perspective.

We could choose to throw a gasket over that traffic jam or bad report card. Or we can take a minute and think through how serious the issue really is. Will it matter next year? Is it something that I can control? Do I need to actually DO anything right at this moment? If your answer to those questions is "no", there probably isn't a whole lot that you should be stressing out about.

One of my favorite questions to ask in times of apparent dire straights is "What's the worst that can happen?" Not because I am tempting the devil or evoking any bad karma. I just want to try to determine the severity of the situation. That way I can have multiple back up plans. I hope for, pray for, and expect the best outcome in any situation... but

I try to have a plan for the worst case scenario as well. It may not work for everyone, but it works for me. That way, if I get rocked by something, I can move to plan B, hopefully unscathed.

Something to think about the next time you THINK you are having a crises or a meltdown. When looked at in contrast to the big picture, does this stuff really matter?

A Wish

If I could have just one wish it would be to stop the world from looking at everything through the I, me, mine lens and channel more energy into compassion and humility.

Rather than telling the world how hard you've trained, how fast you've raced, how lavish your possessions or how exotic your vacation may have been, let's reflect on what we can do, and should do to make "equality" a little more equal, move the bar of acceptance, feed someone who is really hungry, help someone attain the tools of education, help someone feel safe and warm at night, express our love and appreciation of others, and focus our energy into making a difference in the lives of others.

Every single person that you encounter every day of your life is facing some sort of struggle. Some people manage their struggles better than others. And struggles come in a wide variety of sizes and shapes. But everyone is dealing with something. Be that shoulder that someone else needs. Demonstrate a random act of kindness for no other reason than you can.

Have compassion. Show compassion. Live compassion. Be compassion.

Changing one life can change a community. Changing a community can change a society. Changing a society can change the world. We can wrestle and manage our own struggles and still have room in our hearts to reach out to another.

Don't Forget Your Chocolate

OK, I don't mean chocolate as in the cocoa product. I mean chocolate as a metaphor for doing something special for yourself that that fills a void, and satisfies a need, or a sweet tooth. I'm talking about whatever it is that you do that is your "go to" thing to keep you emotionally balanced and on track. Everyone needs something. For those battling disease or treatment, finding that something special that gives you happiness is even more critical to your overall sense of well being. I don't care who you talk to or what you read, the experts should unanimously agree on this point. Keeping your head and heart in a happy, healthy, and adjusted place will aid your healing process.

By now you all know that my chocolate involves some sort of swimming, biking, running, writing, coaching, speaking, working with kids, or mentoring, etc. These are the things that I need. These are the things that satisfy my sweet tooth.

Take them away from me for even a brief period of time and a void is left behind that leaves me restless, uneasy, and eventually depressed. Take them away from me for a longer period of time and the consequences could be worse. However, one of my strengths is the ability to adapt. So, I suppose, if faced with a dire situation, I would be able to find some replacement chocolate, but I prefer not to think in those terms.

You can't plod on day after day dealing with life and all of the issues associated with life without a little chocolate. And it really doesn't matter what form your chocolate takes. Whether you run, bike, rock climb, knit, bird watch, skydive, or cook …. Go do it.

And most importantly, allow yourself to enjoy it.

We all need some chocolate. Find yours.

Looking Back and Moving Forward

So, here I sit. (Quite happily I might add). I live with a chronic leukemia. I manage it – it doesn't manage me. I live above it and not simply with it. And I like to think I am making it count for something. For many years I have always tried to tie sports with philanthropic activities. I am a big fan of doing things for a much bigger reason. When I first started participating in some of my earlier events, I had no idea I would someday have a cause that I could call my very own.

As I look over my shoulder and revisit some of the places this disease has taken me, and the many people that I have been able to connect with, I am reminded that this journey has given me more than it has taken away. I don't think I would say that I truly fear it at this point of my life. I do, however, maintain a healthy respect for it. I also think I have done a pretty good job of navigating through, around, and over the many obstacles this disease has presented.

At the time of this writing, I am again in between follow up appointments with my oncologist. My check up a few weeks ago revealed a slightly elevated white count with a few pronounced lymph nodes. So we once again dialed up a little steroid therapy and I will check in again in a couple of weeks. Ongoing monitoring and occasional maintenance treatment is how this disease is kept in check.

That's ok because I own it and I control it. I will not let it redefine who I am or take anything any from me.

A Cancer Poem

Cancer is so limited…

It cannot cripple

LOVE

It cannot corrode

FAITH

It cannot destroy

PEACE

It cannot kill

FRIENDSHIP

It cannot suppress

MEMORIES

It cannot silence

COURAGE

It cannot invade the

SOUL

It cannot steal

ETERNAL LIFE

It cannot conquer

THE SPIRIT

Author Unknown

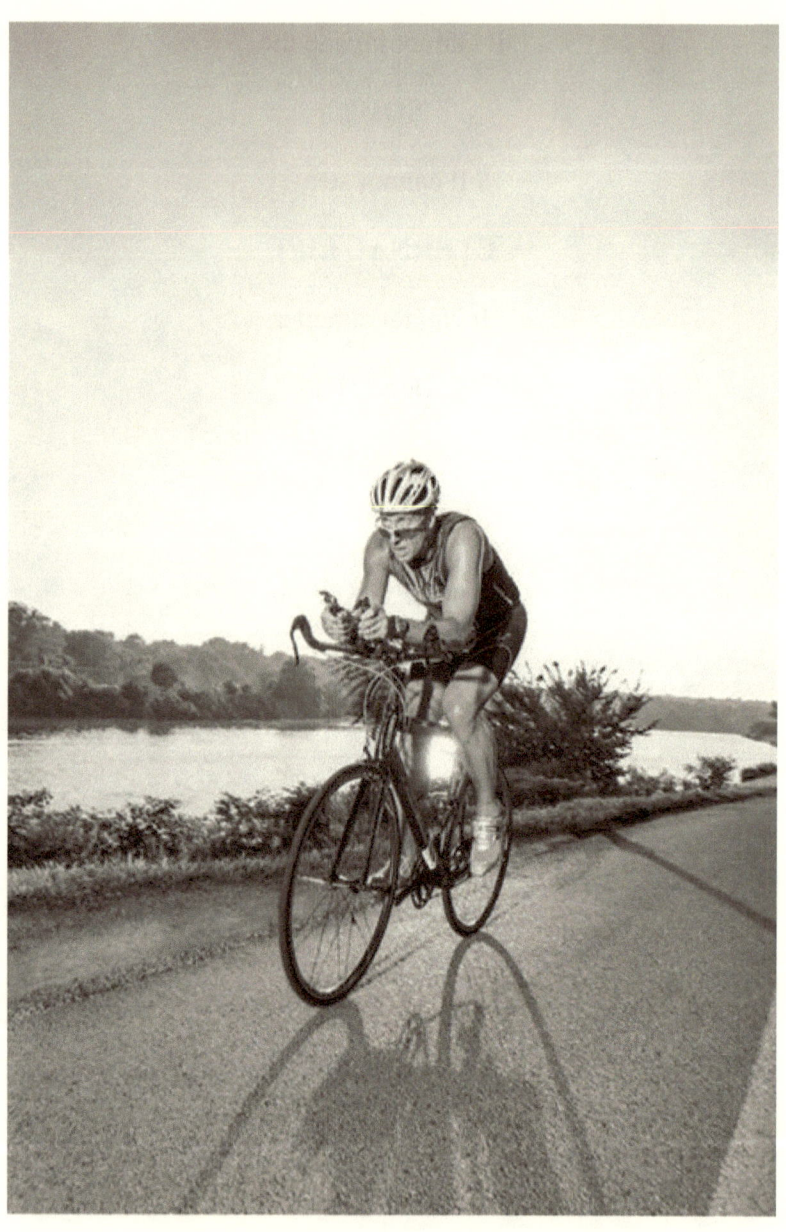

One of my favorite places to train - The Philadelphia Museum of Art loop consisting of MLK Drive, Kelly Drive and Falls Bridge. Photo by Adam Jones.

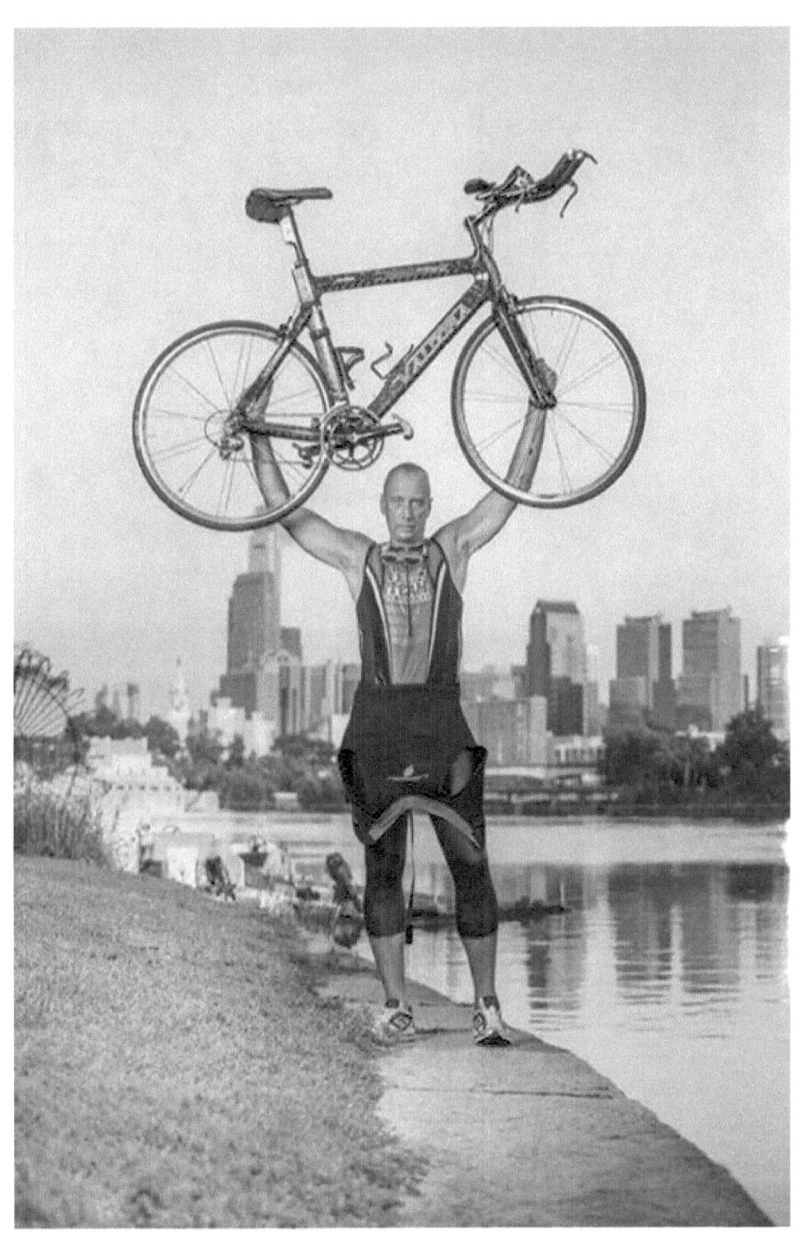

Photo Shoot for a Be Well Philly Philadelphia Magazine piece.
Photo by Adam Jones.

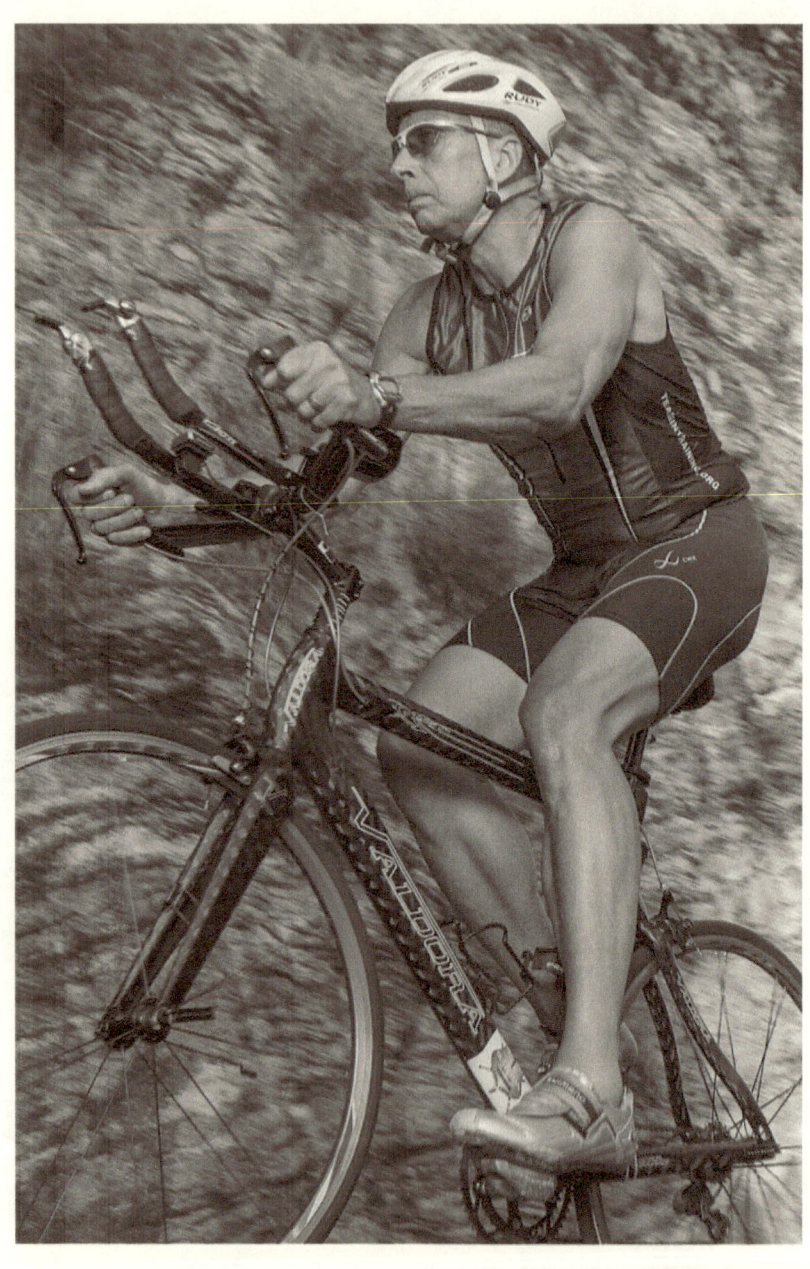

It may look mountainous, but it's actually along the Kelly Drive
path in Philly. Photo by Adam Jones.

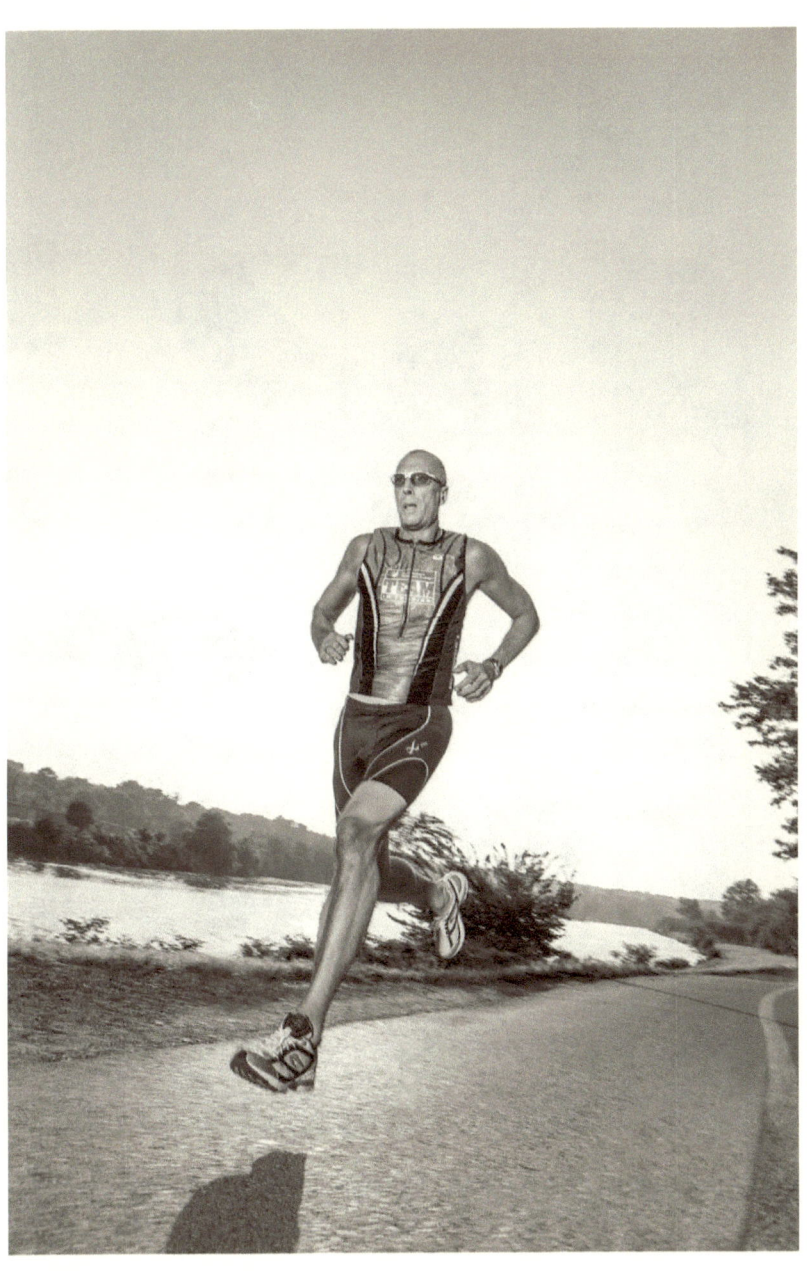

Health and freedom along Kelly Drive in Philly. Photo by Adam
Jones.

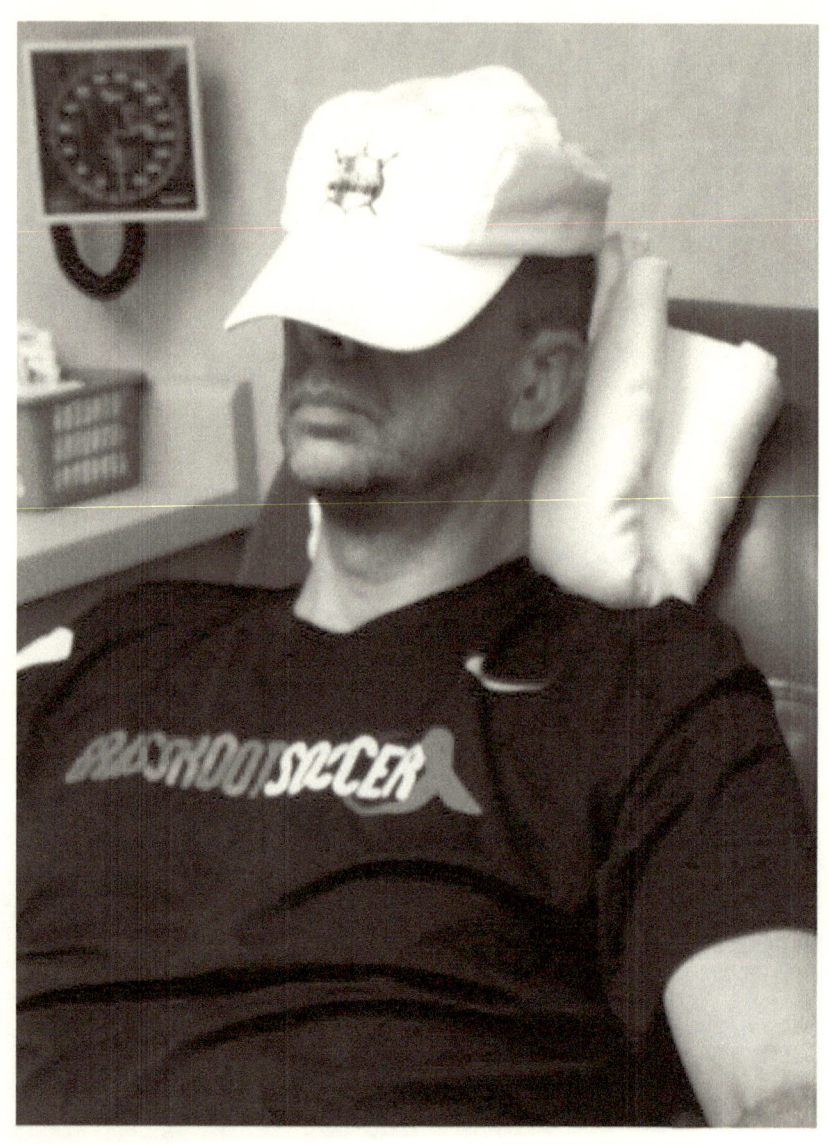

There is always a lot of catnapping happening in chemo.

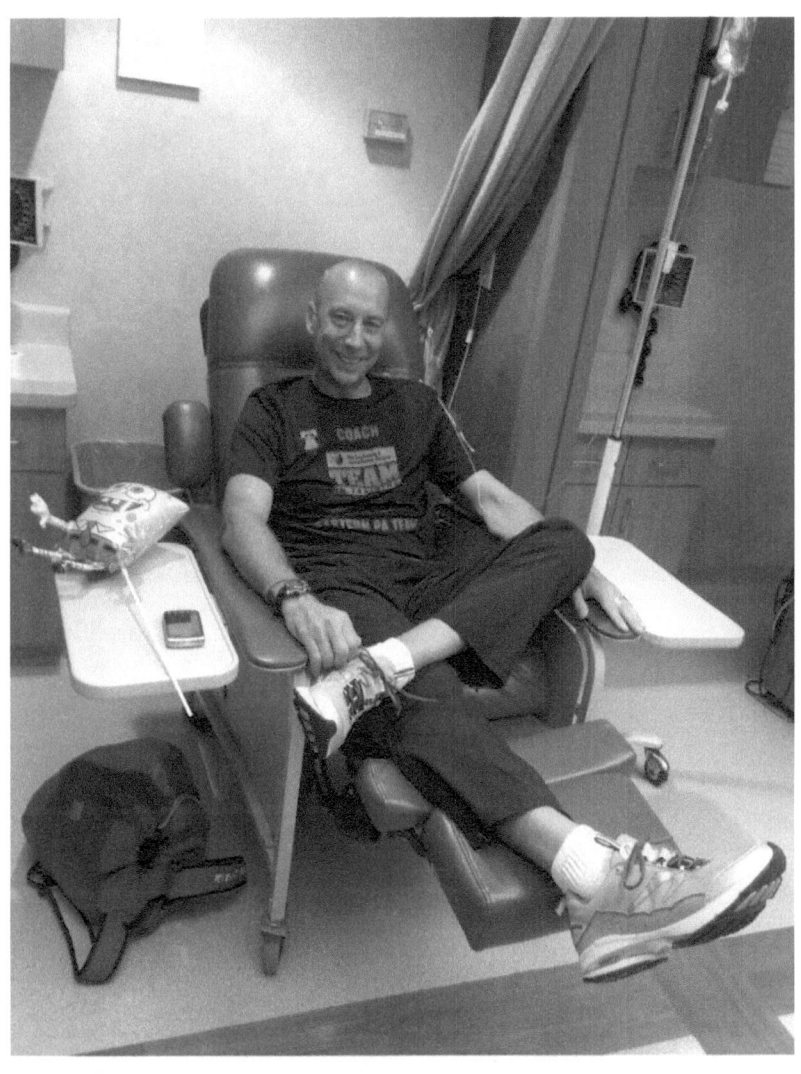

Nothing like a little company from Sponge Bob.

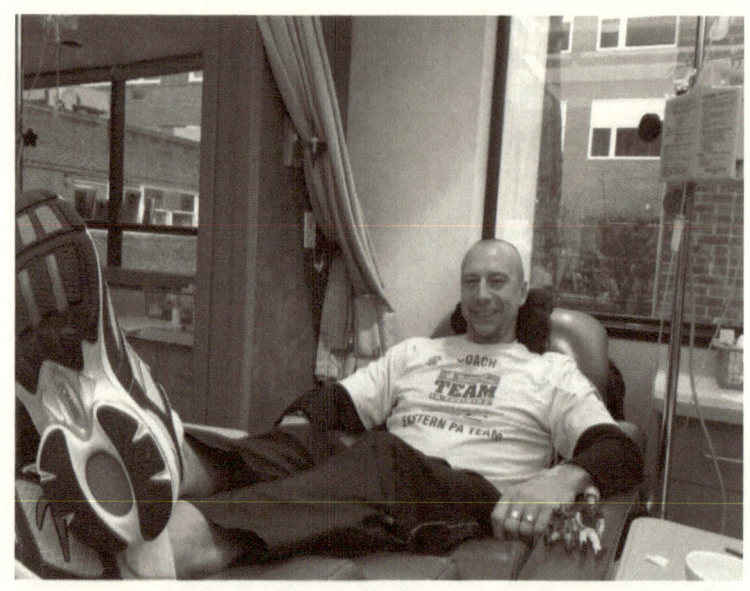

We called for backup for this session. Ironman and Speed Racer answered the call.

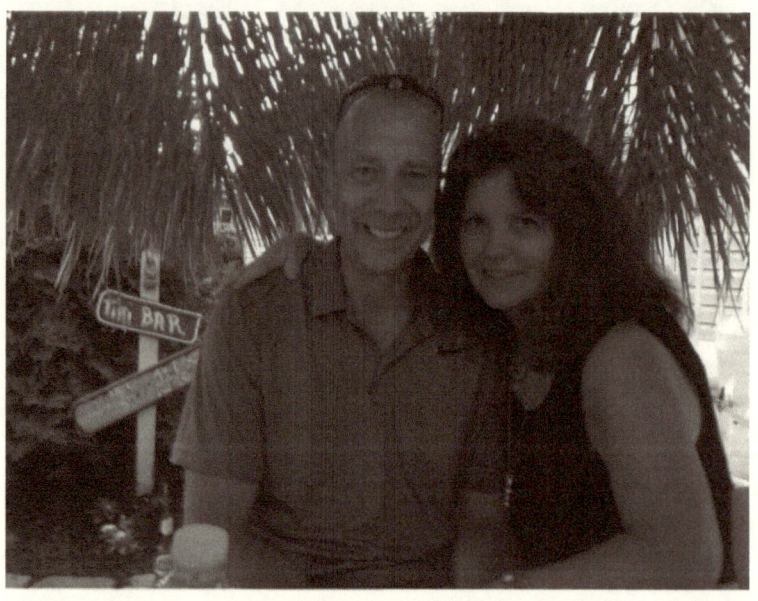

MG and I at our happy place near Ocean City, New Jersey.

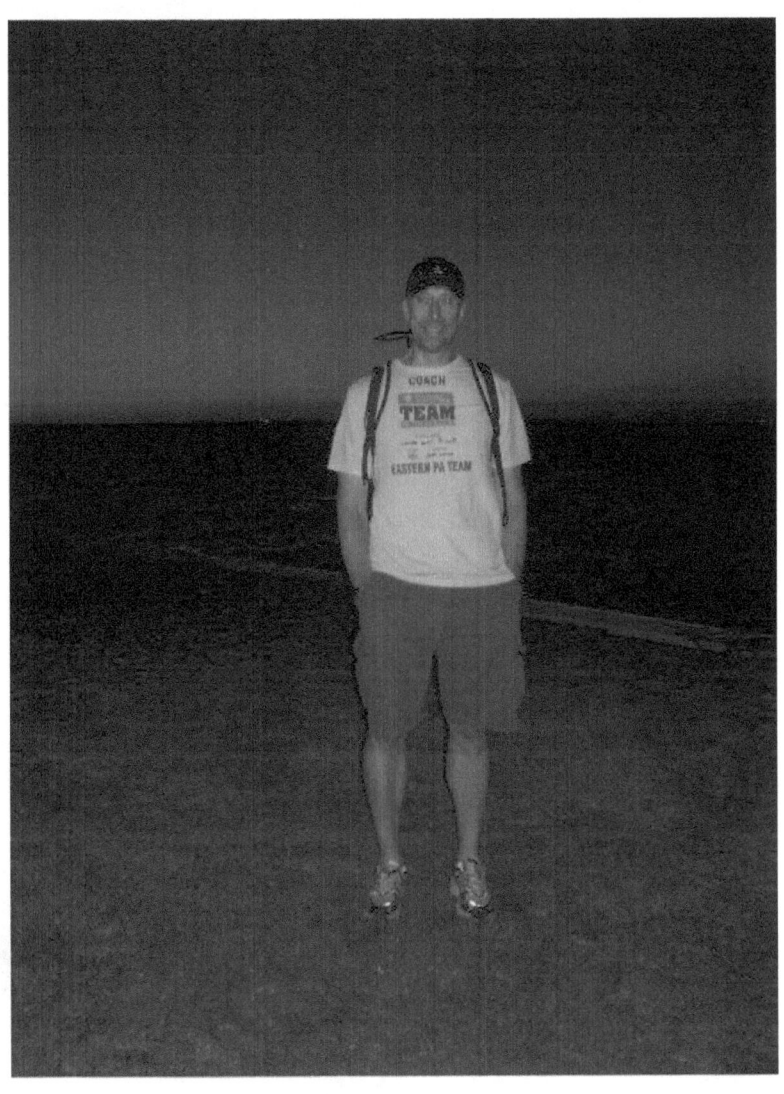

Taking in the dawn prerace calm at St. Anthony's Triathlon in St. Petersburg, FL.

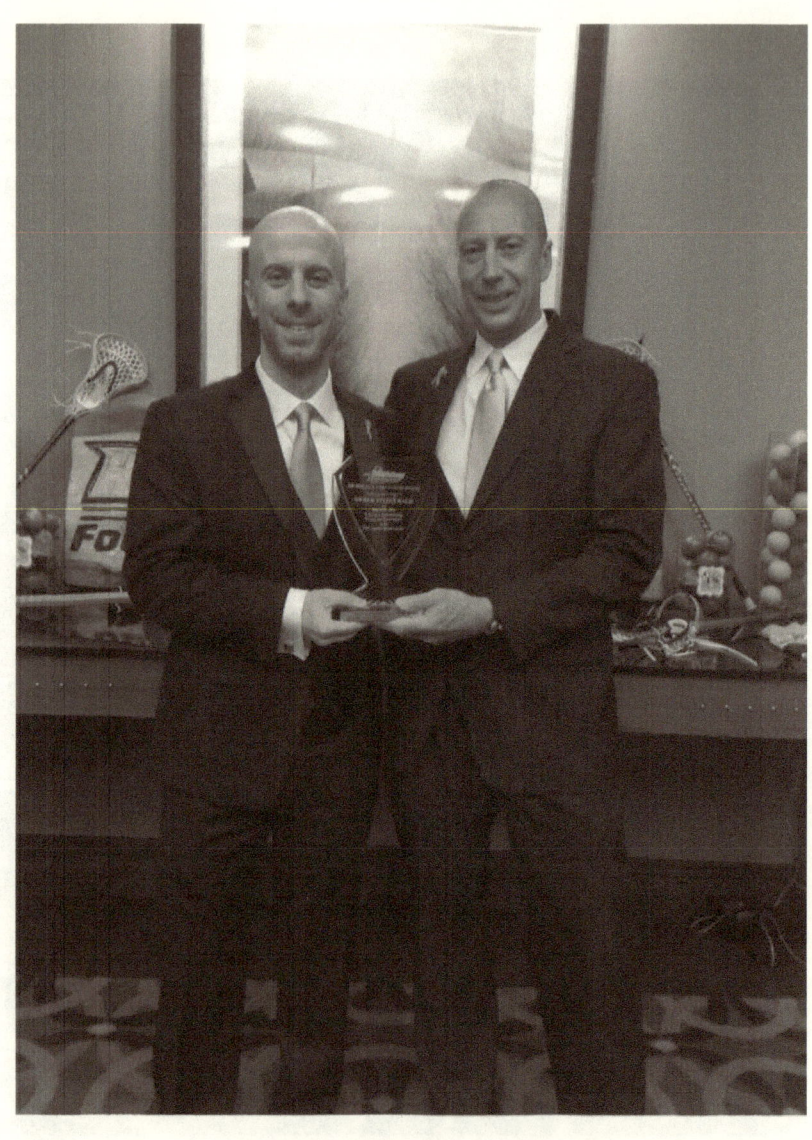

In 2014 I had the honor of presenting the Nicholas E. Colleluori Award to my buddy Derek Fitzgerald. Derek is a cancer survivor, heart transplant recipient, and Team in Training alum.

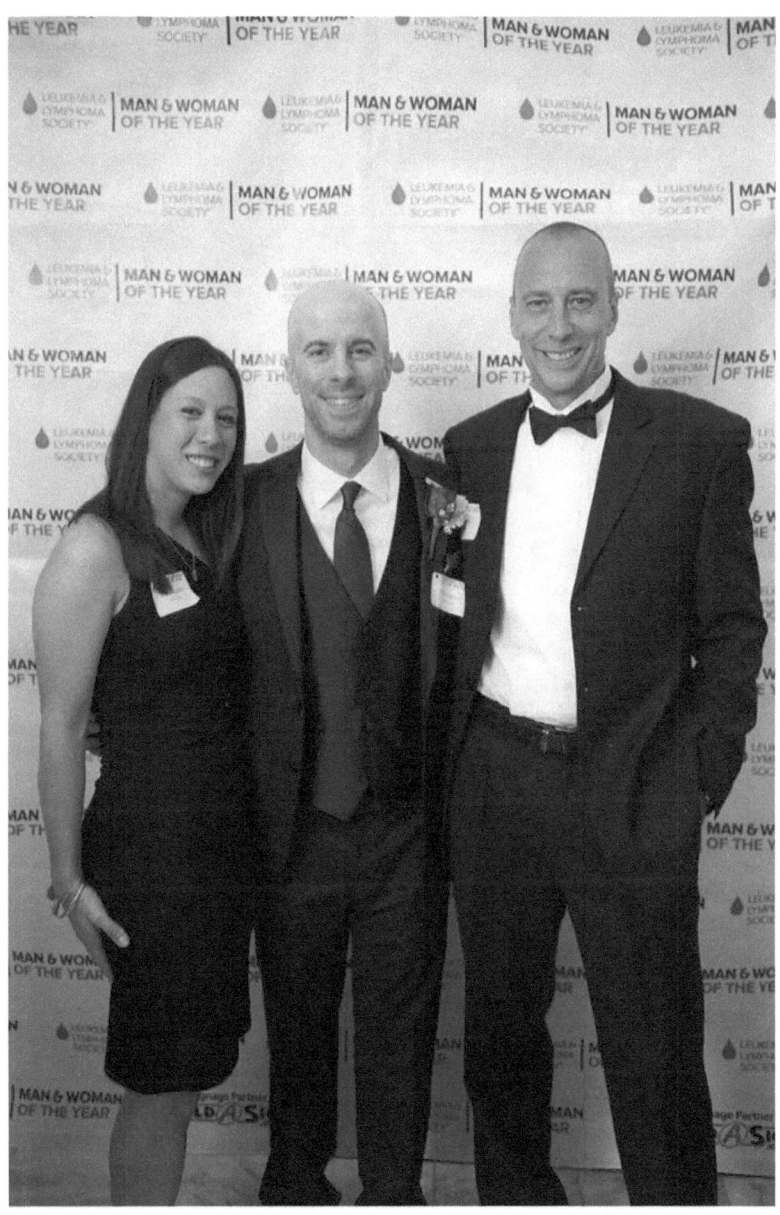

In 2014 Andrea Griffith and I showed support for Derek
Fitzgerald's nomination for The Leukemia & Lymphoma
Society's Man of the Year.

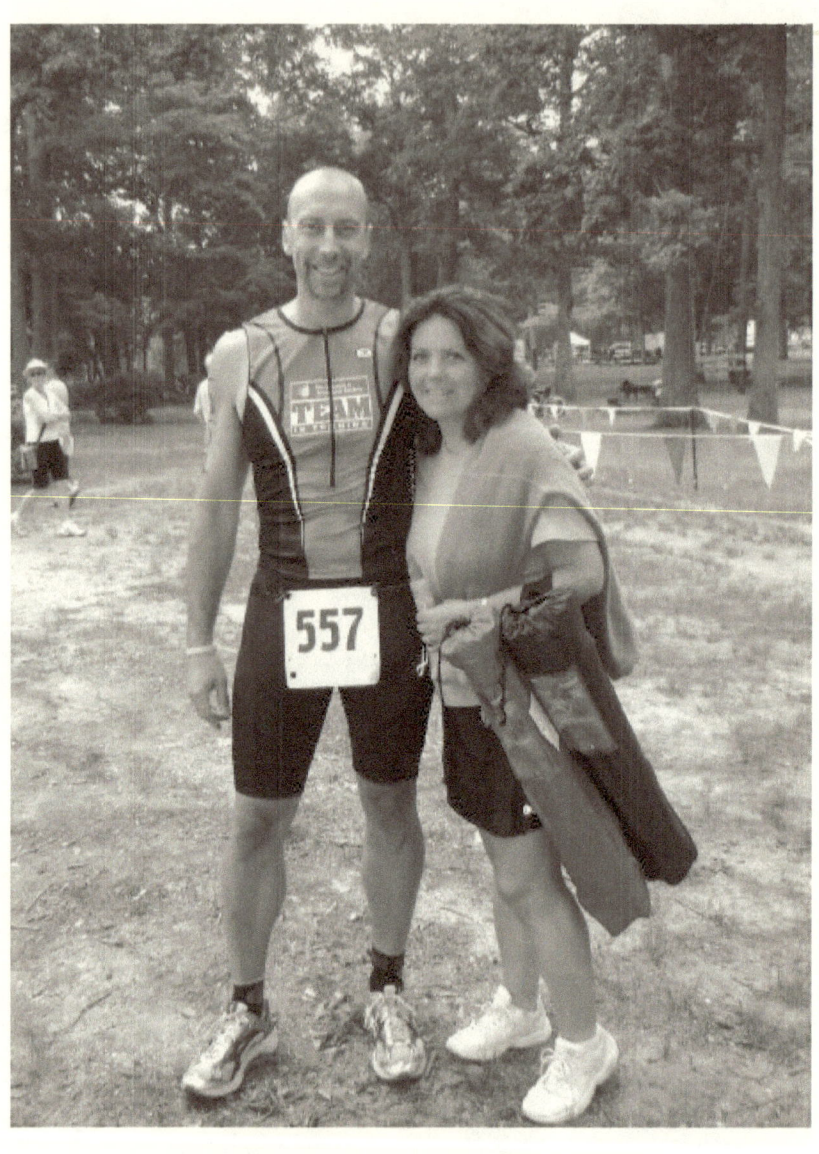

Post race after a sprint triathlon in New Jersey. Mary Grace is where she can always be found - by my side.

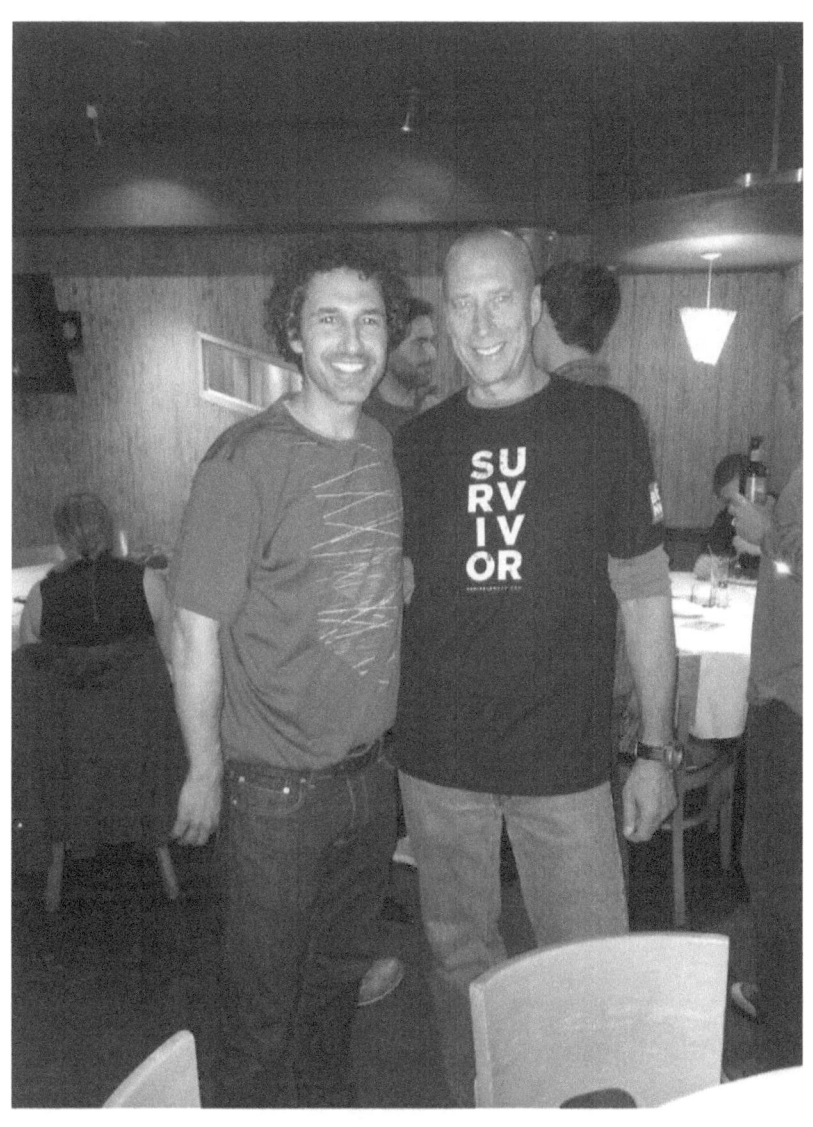

With good friend, fellow cancer survivor, and winner of the
reality TV show SURVIVOR Africa, Ethan Zohn.

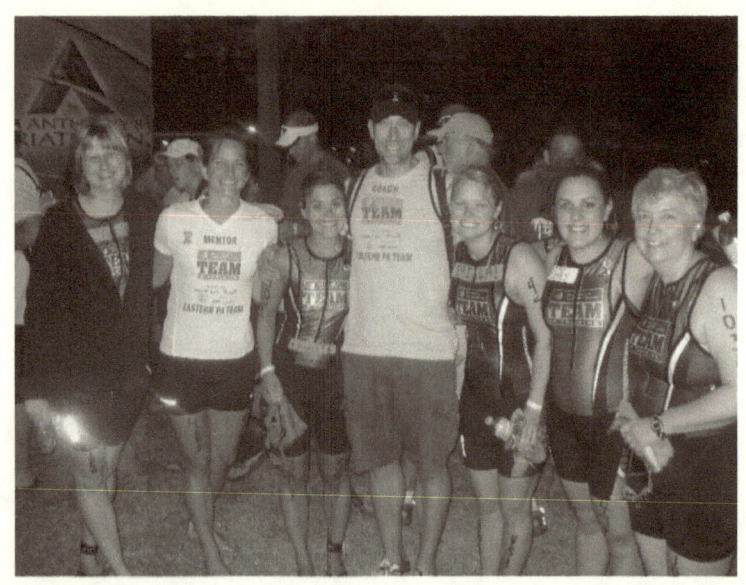

The 2011 St. Anthony's Triathlon Team in Training group rally for some prerace positive energy.

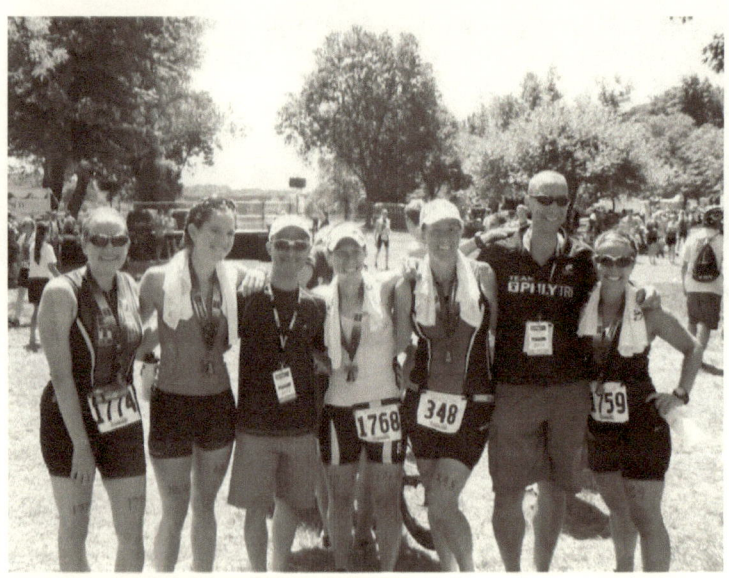

2012 TriRock Philly Team in Training crew celebrate post-race.

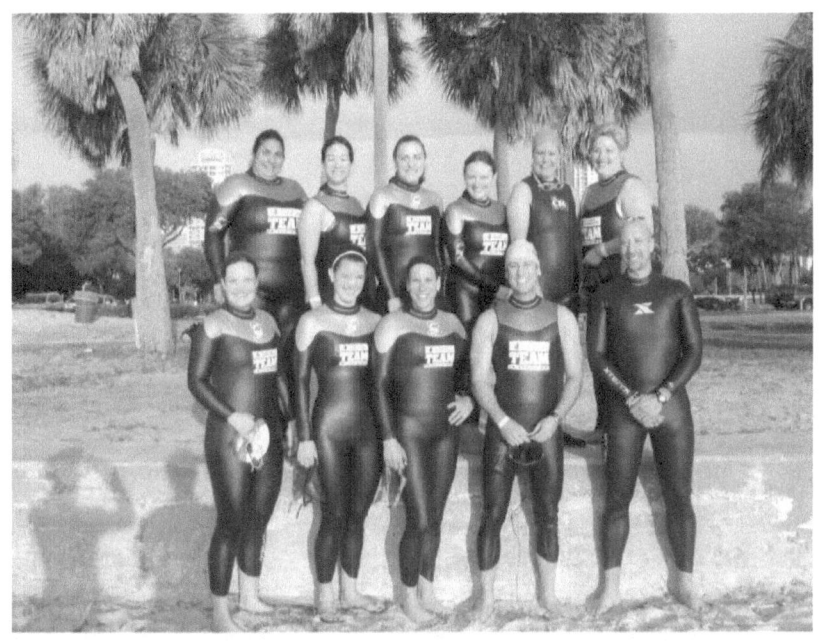

The 2010 St. Anthony's Triathlon Team in Training group
enjoying a prerace dip in Tampa Bay.

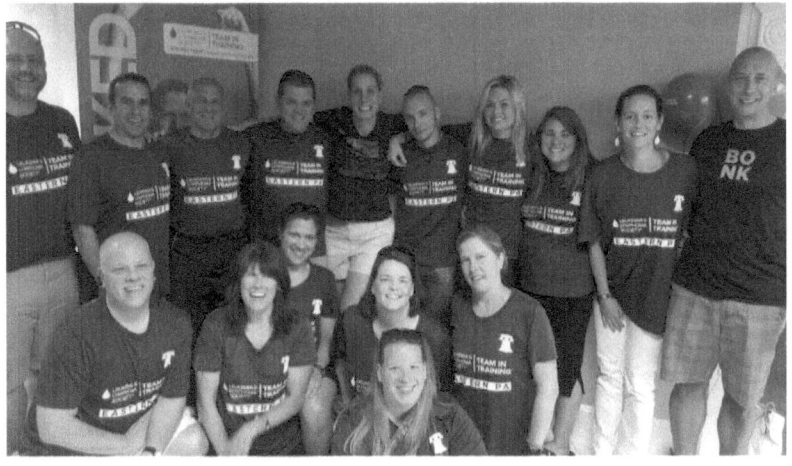

The 2014 TriRock Philadelphia Team in Training heroes gather
for their inspirational prerace dinner.

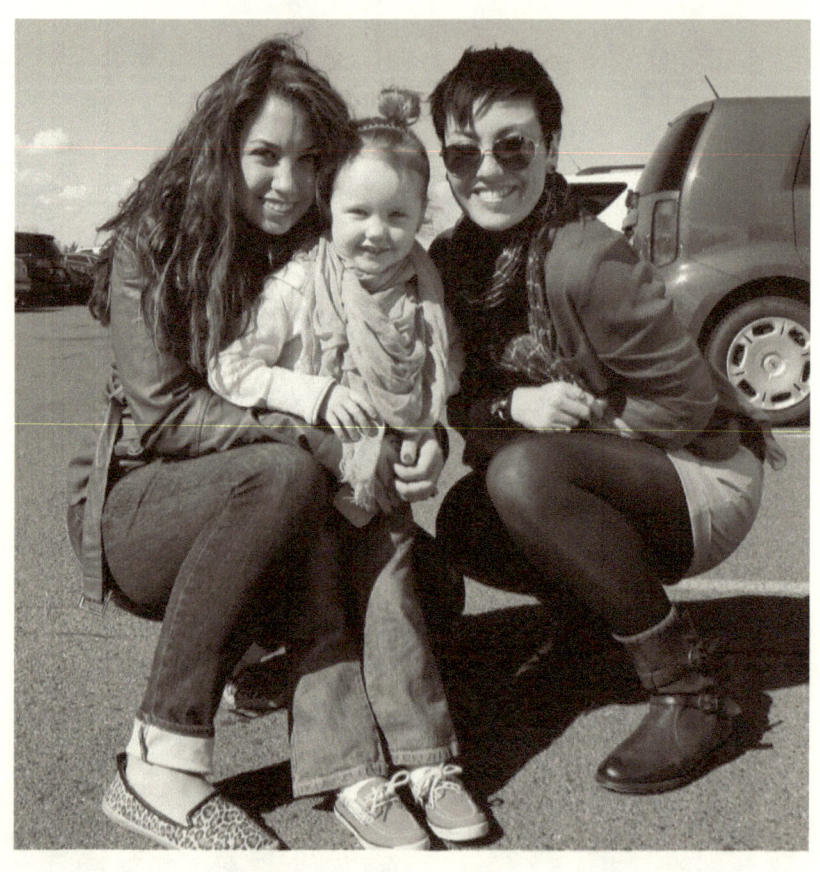

Daughters and granddaughter pride and joy. Danielle Brown with Jennifer Schoener and Brynn.

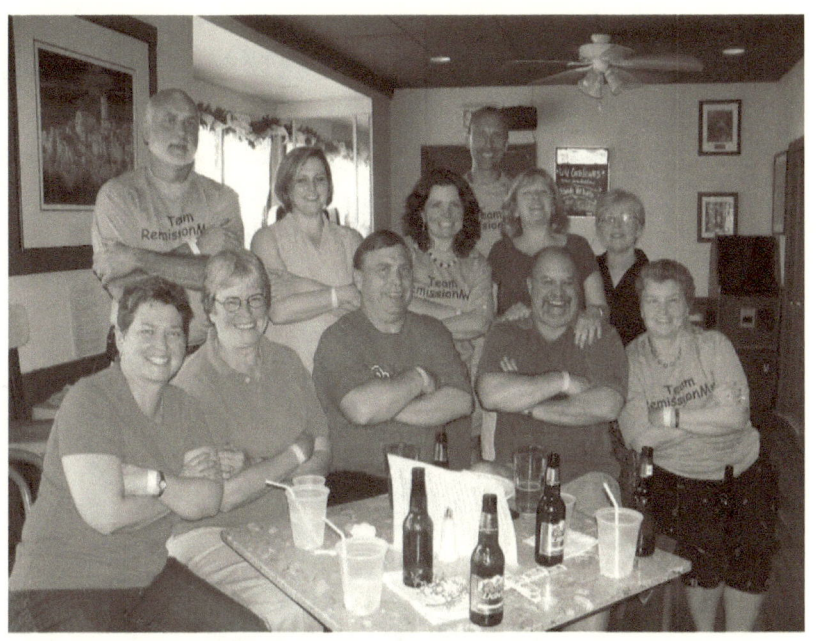

MG's family came out in full force to support this Leukemia & Lymphoma Society fundraiser.

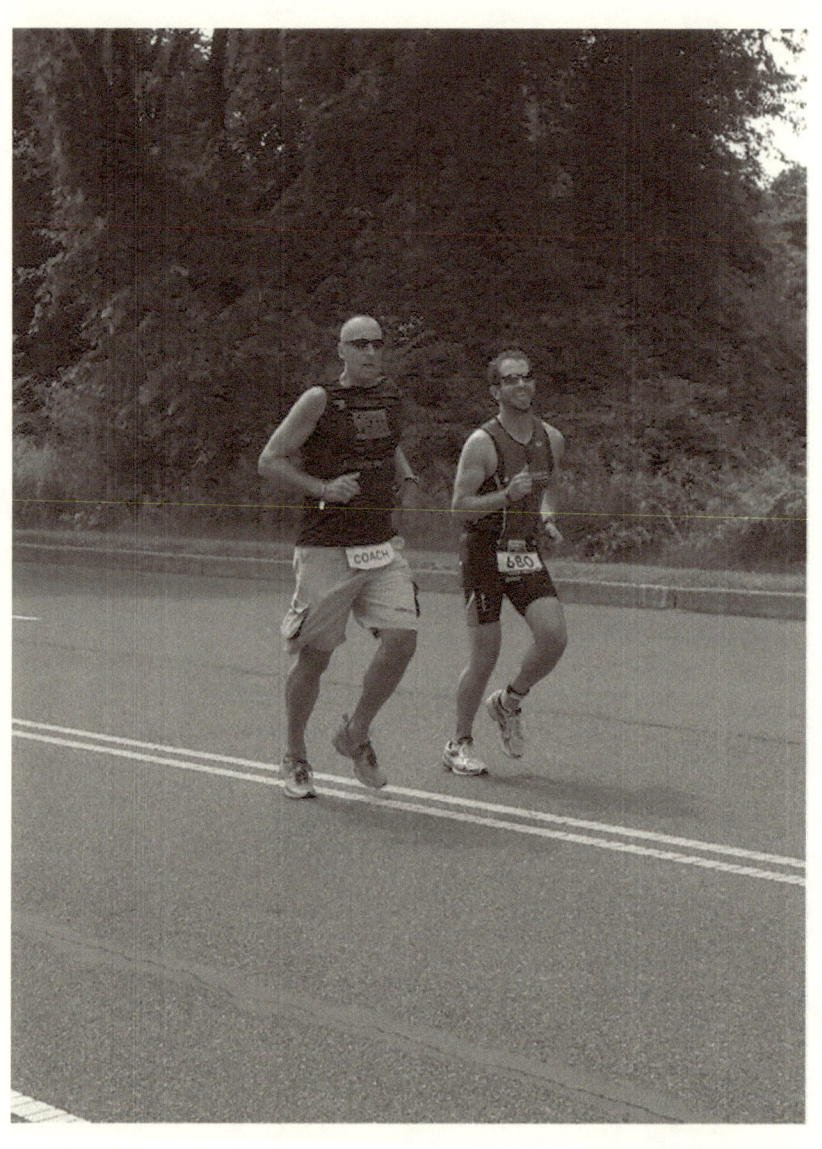

Bringing in Aaron Wagner along MLK Drive at the TriRock
Philadelphia triathlon.

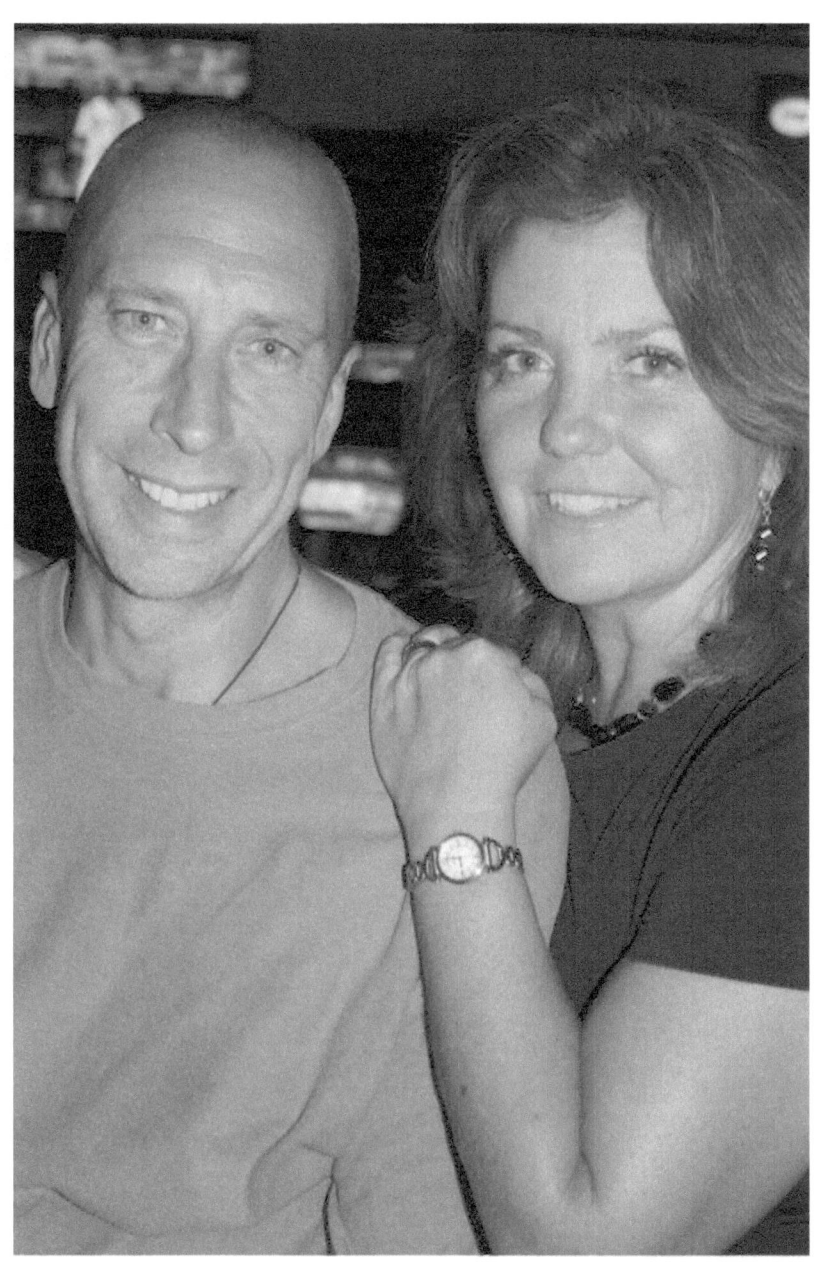

Need I say more?

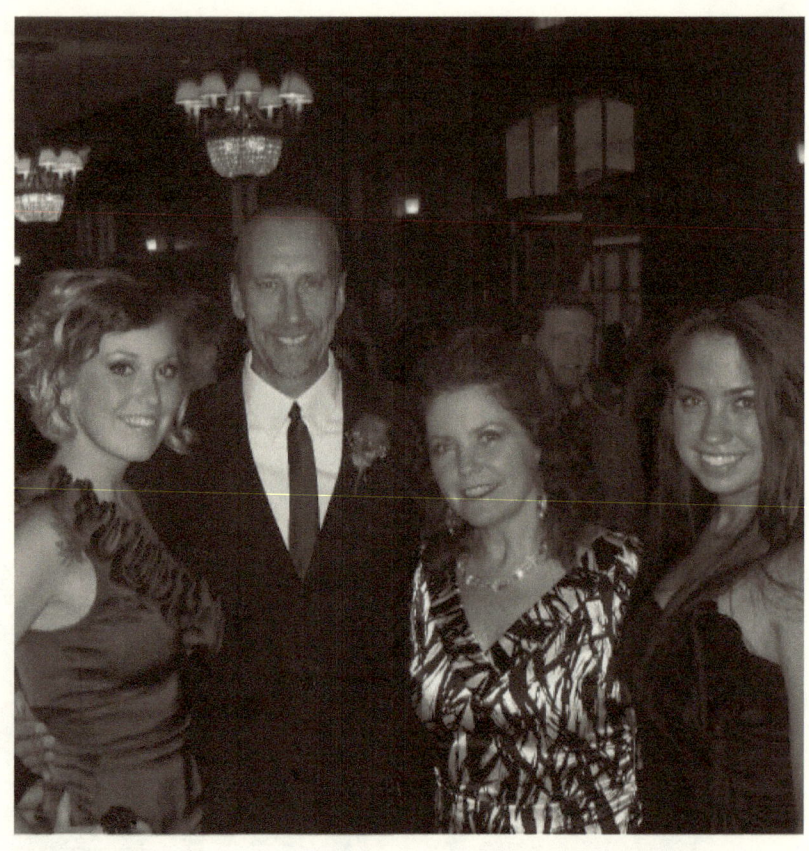

Proud winner of the 2010 Leukemia & Lymphoma Society's
Man of the Year. This never would have happened without an
incredible campaign team and the help and support of my loved
ones, Jennifer, MG, and Danielle.

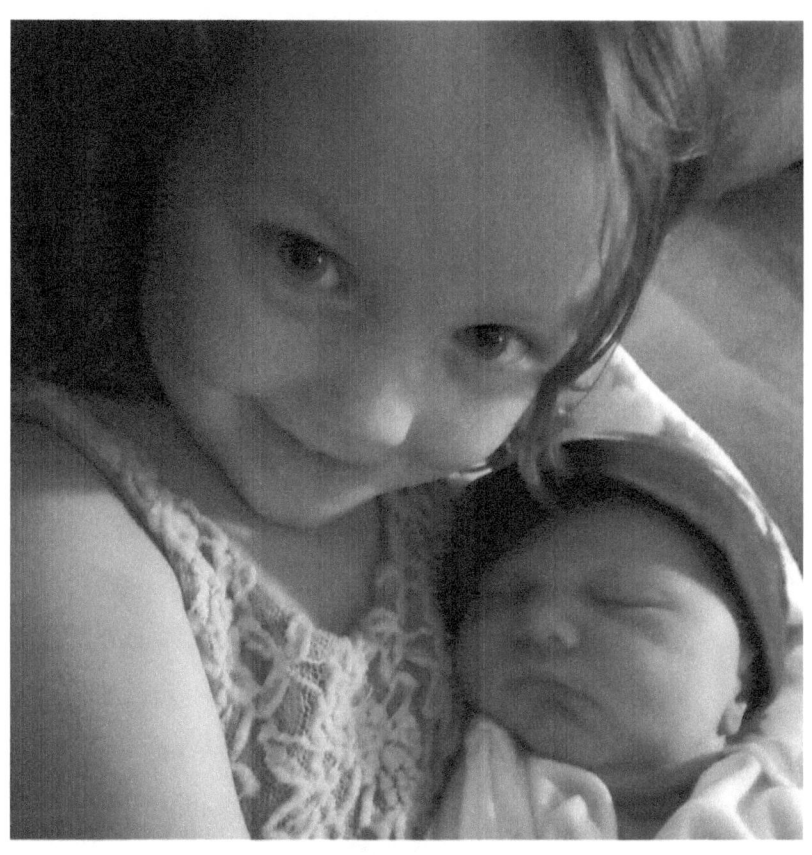

Looking forward to crossing future finish lines with Brynn and our newest grandson Reed.

About Stephen Brown

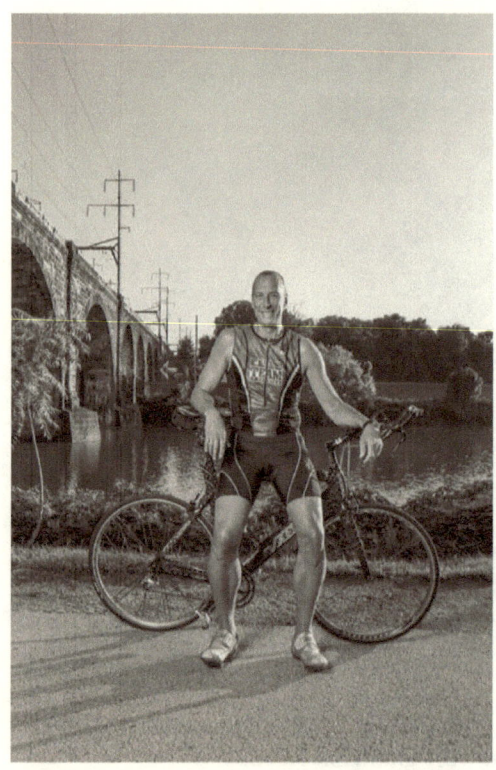

A lifelong athlete growing up in suburban Philadelphia, Steve Brown ventured into the world of multisport racing in the mid-1980s and never looked back. Since that time Steve has racked up countless events of all distances including many marathons and ironman triathlons. Through the years Steve has coached, trained and mentored athletes of all ages from 7 to 70 in varying capacities.

In February of 2006, life threw Steve a curve ball when he was diagnosed with leukemia. Wasting no time, he underwent four rounds of chemotherapy. He maintained his baseline fitness level, often running home from his treatments and quickly reached complete remission.

By July of that same year, he was back to racing triathlons. By September of that year, just 7 months after his diagnosis, "RemissionMan" crossed the finish line of another iron distance triathlon. (2.4-mile swim, 112-mile bike, 26.2-mile run) His diagnosis drew him to the Leukemia and Lymphoma Society's Team in Training program where he now works as a triathlon coach.

In 2006 Brown chronicled the beginning of his leukemia journey with the release of "My New Race". Brown has also written a collection of multisport short stories, articles, and interviews, entitled "The Inner Triathlete ... Forever ablaze". This book is dedicated to Jon "Blazeman".

In December of 2008, Brown released his third book; "50 FIT TIPS". "TIPS" contains 50 fun fitness and motivational tips, reminders, and messages designed to help motivate people and get them moving in the right direction towards better health through fitness.

Brown's fourth collection is entitled "In Search of Center "(Foreword by Ethan Zohn) where he again writes about life, family, disease, and sport.

Steve's writing has appeared in many local, regional, and national print and web based publications and he often speaks to audiences about his journey living with chronic leukemia. He is also a patient mentor to many newly diagnosed patients who has been honored by several organizations for his contributions to the blood cancer community.

To learn more visit www.remissionman.com

About Dave Scott

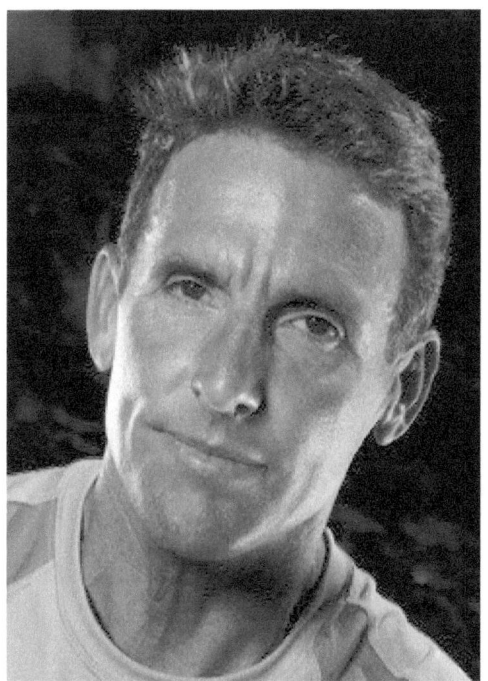

Dave Scott is the most recognized athlete and coach in the sport of triathlon. He is a six-time Ironman World Champion and the first inductee into the Ironman Hall of Fame.

Dave's career in triathlon began with the inception of the sport in 1976. He won his first Hawaii Ironman in 1980 and went on to win again in 1982, 1983, 1984, 1986 and 1987. In 1993, he was honored for his accomplishments in the sport and became the first inductee into the Ironman Hall of Fame. To celebrate, Dave came out of retirement and at the age of forty, after a five year absence from competition, decided to race again. In a stunning and memorable performance, beating out an impressive field of professional athletes – many of whom were in their twenties – Dave placed second overall. This incredible physical and mental feat earned Dave a new nickname among the triathlon community and he has since been known as "The Man".

Dave currently devotes his time educating and inspiring athletes of all abilities and ages, leading sport camps, clinics and races across the country and running his own training group in Boulder, CO. Dave combines years of wisdom, wit and creativity to his passion for helping others. He has been the head coach for Team In Training since 1999, helping to certify TNT coaches nationwide and is actively involved in the running of his business.

Dave Scott, Inc. offers individual and group fitness and nutrition consultations, innovative strength & flexibility e-program exercises, multi-media sport analysis and training tips, video analysis and corporate and tri club speaking engagements and clinics. Dave is based in Boulder, Colorado and greatly enjoys spending time with his three children and maintaining a healthy and physically fit lifestyle.

For more on Dave visit www.davescottinc.com

About The Leukemia & Lymphoma Society

The Leukemia & Lymphoma Society (LLS) is the world's largest voluntary (nonprofit) health organization dedicated to funding blood cancer research and providing education and patient services.

The mission of The Leukemia & Lymphoma Society (LLS) is: Cure leukemia, lymphoma, Hodgkin's disease and myeloma, and improve the quality of life of patients and their families. LLS is the world's largest voluntary health agency dedicated to blood cancer. LLS funds lifesaving blood cancer research around the world and provides free information and support services.

For more, visit www.lls.org

Team In Training is the flagship fundraising program of The Leukemia & Lymphoma Society. Working closely with expert coaches, athletes participate in full and half marathons, triathlons, and cycling events while raising funds and awareness for blood cancers.

For more, visit www.teamintraining.org

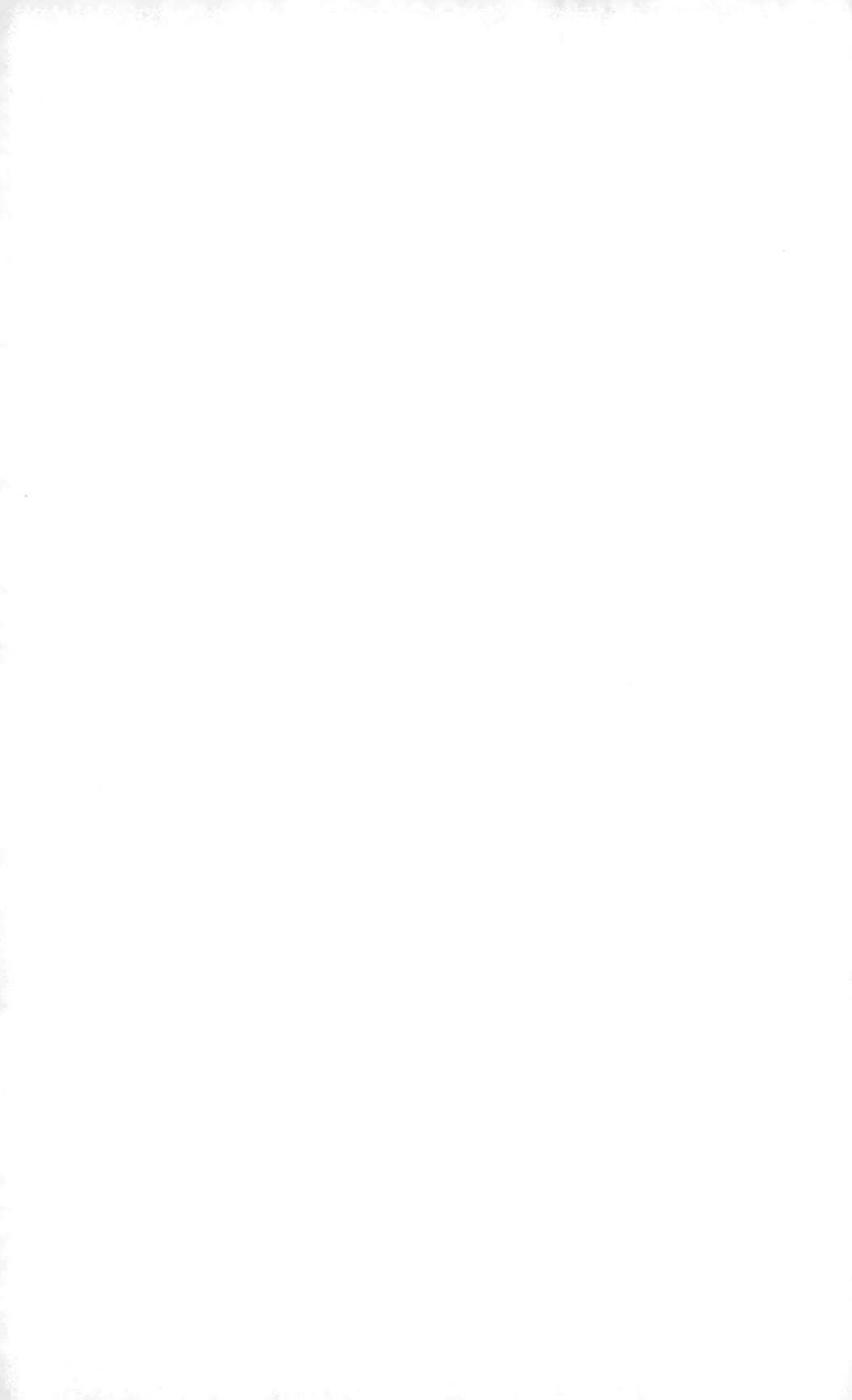